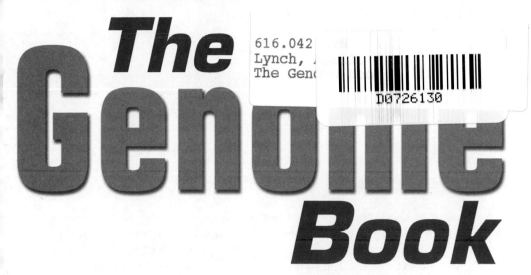

The Genome Book

A Must-Have Guide to Your DNA for Maximum Health

By April Lynch
with Vickie Venne, Genetic Counselor,
Huntsman Cancer Institute

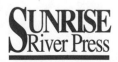
SUNRISE
River Press

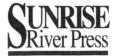

Sunrise River Press
39966 Grand Avenue
North Branch, MN 55056
Phone: 651-277-1400 or 800-895-4585
Fax: 651-277-1203
www.sunriseriverpress.com

Edit by Karin Hill
Layout by Monica Bahr

ISBN 978-0-96248-147-5
Item No. SRP147

Library of Congress Cataloging-in-Publication Data

Lynch, April.
 The Genome Book : a must-have guide to your DNA for maximum health / by April Lynch.
 p. cm.
 ISBN 0-9624814-7-5 (pbk.)
 1. Medical genetics—Popular works. I. Title.
 RB155.L92 2009
 616'.042—dc22
          2007008435

Printed in USA
10 9 8 7 6 5 4 3 2 1

The Genome Book

A Must-Have Guide to Your DNA for Maximum Health

Table of Contents

ACKNOWLEDGMENTS

Any discussion of this book can only begin with my co-author Vickie Venne, who I thank for her scientific eye and dedication to this project. Her expertise, empathy, and good humor make her patients and genetic counseling students some of the most fortunate in the country.

During my many years following the development of human genomics, I've been lucky in finding others who encouraged that interest. My high school biology teacher Stan Ogren showed me that a girl who loved words could also handle science. My editors at the *San Jose Mercury News* understood the importance of genomics in our lives long before most others in the news business, and encouraged me to tell stories of the genomic revolution through the lens of one of its epicenters, Silicon Valley.

I also owe a debt of gratitude to the team at Sunrise River Press, including Dave Arnold, Debby Young, and especially Karin "Doc" Hill. Karin's tireless work on this book has earned her a publisher's version of an M.D.

None of my work on genomics could have been written without the help of the countless medical experts and support groups who've patiently shared their time and insights. I'm especially indebted to the many people with gene-related conditions who have opened their homes and hearts to me. In this book, some of their identities have been shielded, but all their stories hold wisdom for the rest of us. They are true pioneers, and I am constantly humbled by their strength and optimism.

In my career as a science author, I have also been fortunate to work with many leading researchers and doctors, including the dedicated team of genomic experts at Navigenics. It should be noted, however, that the majority of this book was written before my work with Navigenics. The opinions expressed in these pages are solely those of myself and my co-author and do not necessarily reflect those of any past or current employers.

Last, but certainly not least, I am blessed by the support of my husband Colin, whose encouragement kept the words flowing, and our daughter Ava and son Van, whose first years have shown us how something as microscopic as DNA can create new lives filled with unimaginable laughter, joy, and love.

— *April Lynch*

When I was recently asked to give a talk about the genetics of ageing, the title I selected was "Choose your Parents Well"—and I did! Thanks, Mom and Dad, for the good genes and all the support.

On the professional side, Karin Hill and April Lynch offered me an amazing opportunity. Often, scientists struggle to work with journalists, and this book was written when April was at the *San Jose Mercury News*, a newspaper I admire. I marveled at the times that April and I had access to the same information and saw it so differently. April was remarkable in helping me hear language from the public's perspective. Karin Hill was available and supportive—even during her snow days. And this could not have been done without the encouragement of Dr. Saundra Buys and Kathy Schneider—you two are the best.

Since it has been over 30 years since graduation, people ask me how I stay current in this fast-paced field. Teaching is one way. My students continue to challenge my knowledge, and it is stronger for their questions. I thank them.

Writing is another way, and my colleagues help along that path. As we wrote this book, I was responsible for the patient vignettes and pulled from my previous and current clinical experiences as a prenatal, pediatric, and now, a cancer genetic counselor. Many colleagues have discussed challenging cases over the years, and I learn so much from them as well. The cases "From the Genetic Counselor" represent composite experiences, but impart the lessons we have learned when working with patients and their families. For sharing stories and helping with specific genetic questions, thanks go to Jenny Johnson, Becki Hulinsky, Jon Saari, Jeff Botkin, Marilyn Myers, Kristin Peterson Oehlke, Marilyn Ray, Allyn McConkie-Rosell, Sarah Zornetzer, and the many genetic counselors who responded to our listserv. This is the part where I say that these folks are not responsible for any mistakes I might have made along the way!

And my last-but-not-least by any stretch of the imagination is Wendy M. Thanks for keeping me sane.

— *Vickie Venne*

FOREWORD

From the National Society of Genetic Counselors

The routine use of genetic technologies in everyday medical care seems futuristic to some people. But for my colleagues and me, the promises and perils of genetic medicine are part of every single working day. We are genetic counselors; health professionals who provide information and support to people interested in learning more about how variations in their genes play a role in their medical care. We use medical history and family history information to help people find out if their chance of developing a genetic condition is increased. This is called genetic risk assessment. Then we educate people about the risks and benefits of learning more about their genetic information (including genetic tests), provide counseling and support as they make decisions about how much genetic information they want and how they will use it, and aid them in acting on the information they obtain.

A little more than 20 years ago, there were just over 150 genetic counselors working across the country, helping a relatively small number of people with rare or highly specialized problems. What a difference a few years makes! Now there are more than 2,500 genetic counselors at work in the United States. We help millions of people with an amazing variety of medical concerns every year.

This expansion in our numbers and work is part of a much bigger change—the growing incorporation of personal genetic information into many different aspects of health care. We've moved from a more limited world of genetic counseling for more rare disorders, like cystic fibrosis, hemophilia, muscular dystrophy, and Huntington disease, to one where you can use family history information, sometimes with and sometimes without genetic testing, to help you find out if your chances of developing common medical conditions are higher (or lower!) than the average person's chances. Genetic counseling is now available in areas such as cancer, cardiac disease, and mental illness, just to name a few. Furthermore, the number of available genetic tests has jumped from a few dozen, to a few hundred, to more than 1,000 today. Armed with the information you can now get from genetic counseling, you and your doctor can then make decisions about how to best manage your health care in a very targeted way—personalized to you.

These advances mean all of us have new decisions to make. Genetic information is powerful, but it can also be complicated. There are new scientific and medical issues to consider, such as just how much useful information a genetic test will provide. And because your genes are an essential part of your life and your family, they also touch on issues that go beyond medicine. When I help patients make decisions about their genes and their health, we usually talk about their beliefs and values, family relationships, privacy concerns, and many other deeply personal topics. My colleagues and I strongly believe that people need to make their own, informed decisions about if and how to use the genetic information that is available to them in a way that is consistent with their personal and family values, goals and beliefs. Our goal is to provide them with the information and support they need to reach such personal decisions.

Furthermore, we believe that all people should have access to genetic counseling services, provided by an appropriately trained medical professional, before they make decisions about how to incorporate genetic information into their health care. Your genes are part of you for your whole life and are just too important to handle lightly.

Along with the guidance of a medical professional, resources like this book can help you start to think about how to use family history and information about your genes in your health care. This book covers a wide range of health conditions for which genetic medicine is currently in use, ranging from common issues such as high cholesterol to rarer nutritional disorders that babies are tested for at birth. It helps you understand your family history and how genes affect many common health problems, even before you or a family member becomes ill.

To help you understand how to get access to genetics-related health care services, this book also describes the main types of genetic professionals, explains how you can work with us, and points you to reliable sources of genetic information.

The book also talks about the do-it-yourself genetic-testing options that are available. The authors make a consistent effort to point out more questionable forms of this type of care. They also provide you with the information that can help you in making informed choices about using do-it-yourself options, and knowing when a health professional's involvement is especially helpful.

And recognizing the broad effects of genetic medicine, this book goes beyond the purely medical realm. The following chapters include discussion on ethics, privacy and legal concerns, values, and other personal issues, and how each of these issues may have an impact on your decisions about using genetic information in your health care. Each chapter includes a real-life example written by an experienced, highly regarded genetic counselor. Her stories and suggestions give you unique insights into how genetic considerations have played out in the lives of others, and how a genetic professional informs and gives guidance to people in similar situations.

Above all, as you read these pages, I hope you will gain a better understanding of how genes (and the environment!) play a role in health and that you will be inspired to explore how you might use genetic information to improve your own health care. This new age of genetic medicine may seem complicated at times. But I know that many of its discoveries hold the promise of better health for all of us. Welcome to our world! It's an exciting time, for everyone.

— *Catherine Wicklund, MS, CGC*
President, 2007
The National Society of Genetic Counselors
www.nsgc.org

INTRODUCTION

If you'd like to turn one of the biggest scientific breakthroughs of our time into a tool for living a healthier life, you don't need an advanced degree or special access to a research lab. Just remember one idea: Copy the Amish.

It's true that the words Amish and scientific breakthrough don't usually go hand in hand. As a religious community that turns away from many of the trappings of modern life, the Amish don't drive cars, light their homes with electricity, or use telephones. But they do love their children as fiercely as any other parents. And when their kids fall ill, they put their trust in a medical practice that weaves the cutting edge of medicine into the fabric of their lives.

This clinic, set in the heart of Pennsylvania's Amish country, cares for sick children. Its doctors, led by a pediatrician named D. Holmes Morton, treat fevers, visit new babies, and do check-ups. But in taking care of their young patients, this clinic doesn't just rely on regular medical tools and treatments. These doctors use information gleaned from the Human Genome Project and the children's genes to diagnose illness and provide the most appropriate care. These kids aren't part of a research experiment, and they aren't receiving some sort of unproven, risky therapy. They just have doctors who've made genes a regular part of their everyday medical practice, analyzing them when necessary and picking treatments to match. This cutting-edge approach is woven into the rest of the children's care, giving gene science a place alongside stethoscopes, tongue depressors, and the other everyday medical tools that help keep these kids healthy.

The lesson provided by this clinic is one all of us can take to heart. If the Amish can blend new science with their personal values to make their genes part of a healthier life, so can you. This book will show you how to make gene-related decisions with confidence—not just about rare illnesses, but about the sorts of health concerns we all face every day. And we do this in a way that takes into account the fact that we are not just collections of genes, but people.

HOW TO USE THIS BOOK

A plan for good health that factors in your genes—an approach called genomic medicine—isn't a futuristic type of care beyond your reach. Thanks to the Human Genome Project (HGP), which decoded the biological instructions that build a human being, genomic medicine is now at your fingertips. You now have the ability to start turning the Human Genome Project into *your* personal genome project. You don't need to be a scientist or doctor to use the HGP's findings to better understand the instructions that built you, how they can affect your risk for illness, and how they can help you build a lifetime of better health. And you don't need to suffer from a rare inherited condition to find benefits in genomic medicine. This new type of health care goes far beyond unusual diseases or depressing news about untreatable disease risks. DNA information increasingly helps provide insights into many common health issues, including having a baby, fighting cancer, choosing medicines, and calculating your risks for heart disease. Gene-related high cholesterol, for example, is now recognized as one of the most common inherited health problems in the United States. One of the earliest medical exams just about every newborn baby in the United States now receives is a test for genetic illnesses that can be better treated if caught early.

To make use of your genes, though, you need a simple guidebook that helps you start reading and using your personal genomic instructions. The arrival of genomic medicine hasn't been as dramatic as the unveiling of the Human Genome Project in 2000. Instead, new DNA-centered health tests or tools are rolling into use one at a time. An advanced gene test for heart disease risk might be announced one week, while a new medicine to fight cancer is announced the next.

With the amazing volume of health news that hits the airwaves these days, these changes are often hard to follow. And they have to be factored into the reality that your genes affect much more than your health. As an essential piece of your identity, your genome reveals fundamental information about who you are—information that you may sometimes be unsure about discovering or sharing. When it comes to genes, questions of right and wrong are some of the deepest ethical dilemmas of our time, and the choices you make will be deeply personal.

This handbook to your genome and your health takes all these considerations into account, explaining genes and their role in your health from multiple points of view. We cover common health issues such as having a baby, heart disease, diabetes, and cancer. We look at how genes factor into personality, mood, and sometimes even mental health concerns. We point out how your doctors can sometimes use information in your genes to offer you the most effective treatments and medicines. And we also talk about less common gene-linked illnesses—diseases that, while sometimes rare, have served as pioneering conditions in the field of genomic medicine, offering insights that benefit the rest of us.

When it comes to your health, this book can help you:

- Create a detailed family medical history that reveals health risks that may run in your bloodline.
- Discover the DNA tests that are available for many conditions, and decide if any of them are right for you.
- See how DNA and genomic medicine are at work in many common health issues and what options they offer you.
- Find a medical caregiver skilled at blending genomic insights into a plan for good health.
- Learn from other people, whose real-life stories show how genes are involved with real health concerns every day.

Along the way, you'll also find plenty of information that connects your genes and your health to other aspect of your life, helping you:

- Sort through the ethical issues that surround genomic decisions, with ethical considerations discussed throughout the book and a special ethical concern highlighted in each chapter.
- Make important decisions on privacy and health insurance, with practical information on the costs of some genomic care, how insurance companies may use your genetic information, and when laws do—and don't—protect your genomic privacy.
- See how the complexities of genomic care are handled in real life, through stories from a leading gene expert who helps people make the same types of decisions you may find yourself considering.
- Avoid questionable DNA tests or treatments, with consumer warnings featured in every chapter.
- Care not just for yourself, but your entire family, who shares much of your DNA and will likely be affected by any genomic decisions you make.

It's also important to note what this book *doesn't* do. It doesn't tell you that your genes set all the rules for your health, or hold all the answers. Your DNA is a major part of your health, but it works together with your habits, decisions, and surroundings to shape your prospects for well-being or illness. And given that genomic medicine is still an emerging field, you'll find plenty of cases where your genes can't offer much help compared to more established types of medical care. We make those gaps clear, so that you can know when to turn to your genes, and when to look elsewhere.

Even though your genes don't always have the last word on your health, they almost always have something important to say. That's why this time—the era when the deciphering of the human genome can start helping you unlock the secrets of your own—is one to be seized. You can start building a plan for good health that is truly yours, tied to the very essence of the genomic code that builds you. And like the Amish families who rely on their Pennsylvania pediatricians, you can do it in a way that goes beyond the traditions of science and medicine, meshing your genomic information with your values, your family, and all the other facets of your life that determine who you truly are.

To get you started, we turn next to a few essentials—some background needed on how your DNA works, what language it speaks, and how it builds the basics of your body.

CHAPTER ONE

YOUR GENES: ALL YOU NEED TO KNOW

With her warm smile and big-hearted generosity, Josephine Thomas gave no sign of being someone whose body carried a risky genetic difference. A vibrant, dark-haired woman with a loving husband and daughter, she seemed perfectly healthy for much of her life. But one important difference set Josephine apart—a tiny variation in the "instruction manual" that built Josephine's body.

If you could look deep inside Josephine's body and see that difference, you probably wouldn't think it would have very serious consequences. But you'd be wrong. This tiny variation helped create faulty instructions for an important nutritional tool in Josephine's body. Those instructions didn't allow her body to function properly. Over time, Josephine's difference would make her fatally ill.

Josephine Thomas died in 1999, just as the Human Genome Project revealed the details of the instruction manual that builds a human being. Only near the end of her life did she get a chance to understand the tiny difference that had slowly sickened her. She spent her final days urging those around her to read their bodies' own instruction manuals—to undergo a genetic test that would show if they carried the same variation that had harmed her.

You now have the chance that Josephine Thomas did not. In many cases, you now have the opportunity to open your own instruction manual and spot small differences that can have big effects on your health. You can do this long before those differences start causing noticeable problems, long before those differences make you sick. By discovering them early, you can help keep yourself well.

Before you can crack open your own instruction manual or take any steps to protect your health, you need to start learning that manual's language. It is spoken in genes, and this chapter helps familiarize you with the terms and ideas most essential to understanding them.

You may be thinking that gene-speak sounds about as appealing as memorizing a few volumes of tax code. It's true that, most of the time, the world of gene science sounds like a thicket of jargon, strange rules, and odd names. But you don't need lots of complicated vocabulary to help your genes keep you healthy. A few essential concepts will do the trick. You may recognize some of them from a past biology class. Other ideas may be entirely new, reflecting the speed of ongoing gene research.

And don't worry if you're not fluent in gene-speak by the end of this chapter. Even the experts find it difficult to keep up with all the latest developments. This chapter can serve as your cheat sheet, a reference you can return to as needed, whether that is later in this book or during a visit to your doctor's office. With time, this new language will seem routine. If that sounds like a stretch, think back to more than a century ago, when scientists developed a new tool to prevent the spread of infectious diseases such as smallpox. The name they chose for their innovation was vaccination—a strange, unfamiliar term at the time. How unknown is that concept now? Over time, the language of your genes will be just as common.

We'll start with the basics about your genes, and go on to cover the bigger pieces of your instruction manual that you'll need to know to protect your health. Then we'll look at some of the control you wield over those instructions, and cover special considerations for men, women, and ethnic groups. Along the way, we'll also see how each of these parts of the human instruction manual played out in the health—and the life—of Josephine Thomas.

HOW YOUR GENES WORK: THE BASICS

Instruction manuals begin with the letters of the alphabet. Those letters form words, which form paragraphs, which form chapters. Eventually, all those letters and words spell out a complete set of instructions. Your personal instruction manual, the one that built your body, is just the same. It just seems different, because its letters, words, paragraphs, and chapters go by other names—bases, codons, genes, and chromosomes.

Bases: The Smallest Pieces of Your Genes

Bases, or nucleotides, as scientists call them, are the tiny chemical "letters" that spell out the words and sentences that built you. There are only four of them—(T) thymine, (A) adenine, (G) guanine, and (C) cytosine. Four letters may seem too limited to allow your genes to say anything significant. But one look in the mirror offers a reminder that these four letters can spell out some pretty intricate, unique instructions.

Bases do their spelling by lining up in long strings, and then pairing off side by side to form long double rows of letters. This long double chain of bases is called DNA (deoxyribonucleic acid). DNA looks like a curving, twisting ladder, with base pairs forming the rungs that connect the structure across

Did You Know **?**

About three billion base pairs spell out the complete instruction manual for a human being. Printing all the letters of one person's genes in book form would require the equivalent of 200 volumes of the Manhattan phone book, running at about 1,000 pages each.

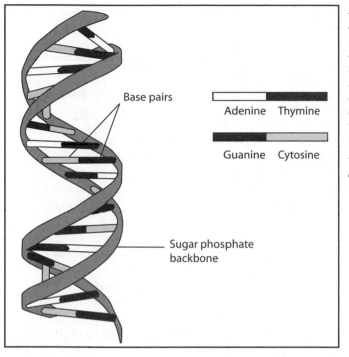

Base pairs

Adenine Thymine

Guanine Cytosine

Sugar phosphate backbone

DNA is made up of bases A, T, G, and C lined up in long strings and paired off side to side to form double rows of letters. This "double helix" design is often described as looking like a curving, looping ladder, with base pairs forming the rungs. The bases are supported by a sugar-phosphate backbone.

the middle. This design is often referred to as a double helix. It gives DNA a distinctive identity—and a unique way to copy itself, which is covered later in this chapter.

Codons: Where Bases Start to Do Their Jobs

Your base letters not only form pairs side-by-side, but also form groups of three. These triplets, or codons, form the "words" in your instruction manual. Each three-letter word—CTA, for example, or GCT—issues the equivalent of a tiny chemical construction command. Your codons tell your body what specific chemical compounds to build where, as well as when to stop building. The piece of information each codon controls is miniscule, but together, as you'll see next, they quickly add up.

Genes: Your Instruction Manual's Basic Work Units

Your codons help spell out your genes. These are the "paragraphs" in your instruction manual—the basic physical and functional units that carry the broader directions for building your body.

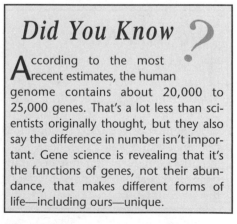

Did You Know ?

According to the most recent estimates, the human genome contains about 20,000 to 25,000 genes. That's a lot less than scientists originally thought, but they also say the difference in number isn't important. Gene science is revealing that it's the functions of genes, not their abundance, that makes different forms of life—including ours—unique.

Each of your genes is responsible for one specific construction function. Genes do that building by issuing instructions for how to make proteins. When we talk about proteins here, we mean something far beyond a food group. Proteins are the basic chemical building blocks that perform most of life's functions. Through the instructions contained in genes, your body produces thousands of different proteins, which help shape everything from your eye color to your blood type.

Genes have clear jobs to do, but they also have some room for flexibility in how they perform them. That's because individual genes often come in different varieties, called alleles. Each allele contains a slightly different ordering of genetic bases. One of your genes carries the instructions that help determine your blood type, for example. But one allele of this gene may come in an A variety, and another in a B variety. The gene remains dedicated to blood type—it just comes in different genetic flavors.

Chromosomes: Packages That Group Your Genes Together

Genes come together to form chromosomes—larger, distinct sets of genomic information. These are the "chapters" in your instruction manual, and scientists have labeled each with a number. For example, the largest chromosome is called Chromosome 1. Almost all people have 46 chromosomes, grouped into 23 pairs.

Almost all your cells follow this pattern, holding 46 chromosomes in 23 pairs. Cells and chromosomes related to gender, though, are notable exceptions. Sex cells, the sperm and egg, contain only 23, for reasons we'll cover a little later on. The sex chromosomes also carry letter labels instead of numbers—the female chromosome is known as X, the male one as Y. And these aren't always an exact match. While women carry a matching set, XX, men tote around an unmatched set, XY.

That variety in XY raises some interesting questions. Why should our other chromosomes carry around a double set of everything else? Why wouldn't just one copy of Chromosome 1 be enough, for example? But there is a reason genes and chromosomes work in pairs. Sometimes, a second copy helps ward off a risk-related variant in the other version. You'll learn more about that backup system later in this chapter.

Genome: Your Entire Collection of Genes

Chromosomes, chapter by chapter, make up your genome, the complete set of instructions that forms you. You'll encounter this term more and more as your genes become a larger part of your health care.

Genes and Your Blood Type

Posted prominently in your medical records, a letter or two spell out how your own mix of dominant and recessive genes has built your blood. The letters list your blood type, and they are a good example of how different varieties of genes and their alleles work.

All healthy human blood functions the same way, delivering oxygen and nutrients throughout the body and carting away wastes. But more than one variety, or type, of blood can accomplish those tasks. Human blood comes in many types, which are distinguished by specific carbohydrates on the surface of your red blood cells. The best-known blood types are referred to by the letters A, B, or O. The A carbohydrate marks what we commonly call type A blood, a B marks type B, and the O in type O equals zero, or the absence of any such carbohydrate.

Each variety arises from the same section of DNA, the *ABO* gene, found on Chromosome 9. The A, B, and O are each one of the gene's alleles. You inherited two alleles of the *ABO* gene, one from each of your parents.

Dominant and recessive genes set the rules about which alleles determined your blood type. A and B are dominant alleles over recessive O. In an interesting twist, neither A nor B rules the other, a phenomenon called co-dominance. When people carry these two equally powerful alleles, they have type AB blood. Type Os, however, have inherited two recessive O alleles. Otherwise, the presence of an A or B allele would outweigh their lone O.

Here's how those alleles add up to the most common blood type combinations:

O + O = Type O
A + O = Type A
B + O = Type B
A + A = Type A
B + B = Type B
A + B = Type AB

Why would human blood come in all these different varieties? As with many gene differences, the alleles for blood type likely arose to help keep people healthy. Some blood types appear to be better than others at fending off particular diseases. Those with an A marker on their red blood cells appear to have more resistance to cholera, for example. Type Os may carry more resistance to malaria.

In our age of modern medicine and blood transfusions, though, blood type alleles also can also sometimes bring serious health risks. Alleles make it tricky to mix different types of blood. Since type O blood lacks a type carbohydrate, anyone can receive it. But As can only receive blood from As or Os, Bs from Bs or Os, and Os from Os alone. Mixing incompatible blood types can be very dangerous, so knowing your blood type is an important part of protecting your health.

Your As, Bs, or Os, of course, don't tell your whole story. Everyone's blood type is marked by many other features, including a positive (+) or negative (-) sign. This symbol relates to another gene-driven blood factor called Rh. Rh factor is discussed more in Chapter 4.

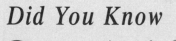
Genomic science, for example, usually refers to studies of the human genome. Genomic medicine refers to any health-related use of gene information. Genomic medicine is different from another term you're probably familiar with, genetic disease, which refers to illnesses that are passed from parent to child. Genetic disease is just one part of genomic medicine.

As your full set of genetic information, your genome sits inside almost all of your body's basic work units, your cells. Cells contain a core called the nucleus, which holds the genome and gives it a sort of operational headquarters. From the nucleus, genes issue instructions for proteins, which then form and direct most cell functions. While almost all your cells contain a full copy of your genome, not all genes issue instructions in every cell. The genes that dictate how your liver functions, for example, don't get too involved in growing you a new eyelash.

All those genomic pieces direct your body's form and function, day in and day out, from the moment you were conceived. They help you digest a bag of popcorn, talk on the phone, and heal a burned finger. Sometimes, if they don't function quite precisely, they can also affect your health. To get a sense of how that happens, let's go back to Josephine Thomas.

Josephine had the typical 46 chromosomes—23 pairs—including one pair called Chromosome 6. That chromosome's 1,500 or so genes include one called the *HFE* gene. This gene makes an important protein related to nutrition, regulating how much of the iron from the food you eat flows into your cells. You need some iron for good health, but too much can cause an illness called hemochromatosis, or iron overload. This damaging condition can, over time, ruin your liver and harm your heart. If left untreated for years, often because it is overlooked or misdiagnosed, hemochromatosis can kill you.

Hemochromatosis Facts

• Among Caucasians of northern European descent, about 1 out of every 8 to 12 people is a carrier. An *HFE* mutation is one of the most common among this population group, making this group the most likely to benefit from an *HFE* genetic test.

• Symptoms include joint pain, fatigue, darkening of the skin, heart problems, and liver problems.

• While the *HFE* mutation is the most common cause of hemochromatosis, the condition sometimes has nothing to do with genes. Other causes include blood transfusions, liver disease, and overuse of iron supplements.

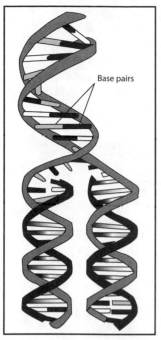

Base pairs

Genes reproduce themselves by splitting (or unzipping) their double helix of DNA into two halves. This results in two single, unmatched sets of base pairs, both of which quickly bond to new strings of bases, forming two new separate copies of the original gene.

The HFE protein protects most of us from iron overload, thanks to an important codon on the *HFE* gene—TGC. This string of three bases helps ensure the creation of a fully functioning HFE protein that keeps iron levels under control. In most people, that little TGC helps make sure that you get just enough iron from the spinach in your scrambled eggs at breakfast, and that the rest gets flushed from your body.

In Josephine Thomas, the set of instructions for the HFE protein was misspelled. Her instructions didn't read TGC. They were one letter, or one base, off. Instead of a G, her codon held an A.

That one change, that TAC where TGC should have been, was enough to disrupt the normal functioning of her *HFE* gene. In Thomas and others who share her misspelled codon, this misplaced A gives them an HFE protein that can't control iron flow correctly. In Josephine Thomas, years of iron buildup slowly damaged her liver, opening the door to the liver cancer that eventually claimed her life.

How could a difference like that get into a person's instruction manual? And why couldn't the error be fixed somehow, by the body itself or by medical treatment? The answers start with the ways genes copy themselves, sustaining you and giving rise to new life along the way.

Your Body's Internal Copy Machines

Your genome is more than just an instruction manual for making proteins. Your DNA also carries the instructions for making more of itself.

Guided by the instructions in your genes, your cells constantly copy themselves by dividing into new cells. Gene scientists term these cells somatic cells. These newly minted cellular replicas let you grow as a child and thrive as an adult, replacing worn-out cells with fresh ones. But as they recreate themselves, your cells and genes can only work with what they've got. They make copies of the instructions for all your best gene features. But they also replicate instructions for parts that might not work as well. And sometimes, in the midst of all that copying, an error is made.

Understanding how your genes recreate themselves is an essential part of helping your genes keep you healthy. Here's how it all works.

How Genes Make New Genes—and New Cells

When it is time for some of that cellular regeneration, the process starts with the double helix of DNA coiled inside almost all your cells. In the cell to be copied, your DNA first splits, or unzips, into two halves, creating single, unmatched sets of base pairs. Since bases like to stay in pairs, new bases then bond to the unzipped strands. This quick sequence of unzipping and rebonding leaves you with two new copies of your genome. A new cell forms around each of these new genomes, resulting in two complete new cells.

This process happens at wildly different rates throughout your body. Many human brain cells are formed early in life and live for decades without dividing again. Cells that form the linings of your body, such as skin cells, regenerate more rapidly, dividing about once a day.

How Genes Make New People

The copying process is a little different for cells that make babies. Since a full genome consists of chromosome pairs, a new child needs only half a genome, or 23 chromosomes, from each parent. That is why sex cells have the difference we mentioned earlier—sperm and eggs carry only carry 23 chromosomes, not 46.

Sperm and eggs wind up with a half set of chromosomes because they arise from germ cells. Here, germ refers to new life, not microbes that give you the flu, and the term describes cells that give rise to life through a special way of dividing. The process of making these cells halves the number of chromosomes from 46 to 23. The process also shuffles bits of DNA, resulting in sperm and egg cells containing genes that read a little differently from the originals, lined up in a half-set of 23 chromosomes ready to find a match and make a new person.

Mom or Dad: Whose Genes Decide How Baby Develops?

Once those 23 and 23 add up to 46, though, there's still one issue to sort out. Whose set of genes makes the rules—Mom's or Dad's? Dad's germ cells decide whether a baby is a boy or a girl. But when it comes to other characteristics, the rules depend on whether one of the two genes in this new set carries more clout than the other. In the rules of the genome, this power dynamic is referred to as dominant or recessive. Here is how it usually plays out:

- If one gene is dominant over the other in its pair, the dominant gene sets the rules.
- If neither gene in a pair is dominant, usually because two recessive copies have been inherited, the recessive instructions get to do the work.
- If you inherit a dominant and recessive copy of a gene, the dominant version does the work, but the recessive copy remains in your genome and can still be passed on to your children.

A person with only one copy of a recessive gene is called a carrier. Many carriers often have no effects from their single gene copy. In some cases, however, carriers may face some additional health risks from their single copy of a health-related gene difference. Hemochromatosis carriers, for example, sometimes have elevated levels of iron in their blood. More of these types of risks are covered as we discuss specific health conditions through this book.

Children of carriers may also face some additional health-related risks. If a carrier happens to have a child with another carrier, there is a chance their child will inherit two copies of the recessive gene and develop a genetic illness. And since children of carriers can also inherit one copy of the affected gene, they can also become carriers and pass the recessive gene down the family bloodline.

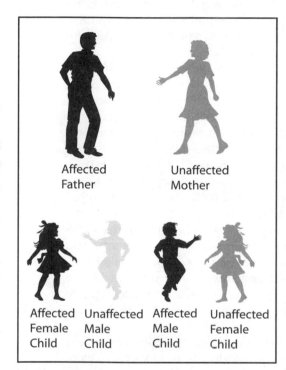

Affected Father   Unaffected Mother

Affected Female Child   Unaffected Male Child   Affected Male Child   Unaffected Female Child

In dominant genetic disorders, if one affected parent has the disease-linked gene, there is a 50% chance that each child will inherit the disease-linked gene and the disorder.

In the Thomas family, this dynamic played out from generation to generation. The *HFE* difference that Josephine inherited is recessive. To receive two copies of the recessive gene and develop hemochromatosis, Josephine had to have one copy from each parent. Neither of them knew they carried the *HFE* mutation.

Josephine's inheritance, and her illness, reflected only a dose of genomic bad luck. If either one of her parents had given her a normal version of the *HFE* gene, that one normal copy would have been enough to override the misplaced A in her *HFE* gene. But with two recessive copies of the gene, Josephine's misplaced A spelled out the only instructions her body had to follow.

Conditions such as Josephine's, arising from a pair of recessive genes, are referred to as recessive disorders. However, diseases can also arise from a single, dominant gene. These diseases are referred to as dominant disorders. The dominant or recessive nature of a disorder affects a parent's chances of passing it on, as well as a child's chances of inheriting it.

Why Genes Come in Many Varieties

Why are there so many different versions of genes? Between alleles, dominant genes, recessive genes, the genome's copying process might seem a little too error-prone for comfort.

In reality, most of the variations in the human genome work to your benefit. Gene changes give our species its enormous diversity and resilience. More genetic variety means each of us has a smaller chance of inheriting two risk-related copies of any particular piece of DNA. And many gene variations have few serious effects. Brown eyes may be a different color from others, but they can see just as well as hazel, green, or blue.

Most gene varieties arise from a process called mutation. To most people, that word often sounds scary. Mutation and mutant have come to equal disease, or evoke images of wart-covered monsters from sci-fi movies. But at its most basic level, a mutation is simply a change to the sequence of bases appearing in the DNA inside a cell. Many mutations are harmless. Only some trigger illness, and those that cause serious illness are very rare. Nor do mutations make up most of your genome. All people share more than 99 percent of the same DNA.

The DNA that sits within that one remaining percentage of difference is what makes us distinct from each other. These gene variations are called polymorphisms. They're responsible for many of the differences you see among people every day, such as hair color. The smallest differences, involving just one base letter, are called single nucleotide polymorphisms or SNPs, a term pronounced "Snips." Gene scientists believe about 10 million SNPs exist in the human population, affecting all sorts of features and functions. And as the single letter change in Josephine Thomas's body shows, SNPs can sometimes have powerful effects on your health.

How do these variations happen? Mutations can occur in any gene inside any cell of your body at any point in your life. To start understanding the most common form of mutation, think about the last time you tried to copy a passage out of a book, either on the keyboard or by hand. No matter how careful you were, you probably made a mistake. Maybe you reversed the order of a couple of letters or words by accident, or spelled something wrong. When you make copies, you may make inadvertent changes.

The same holds true with DNA. Mutations can arise when germ cells make copies of their chromosomes before dividing to form sperm or eggs. The process usually goes smoothly. But sometimes, DNA makes a mistake. Maybe a base winds up in the wrong place, or gets left out. Or perhaps extra copies of some bases are made, or a long stretch of a chromosome winds up rearranged.

Such serious changes are rare. Scientists have found that DNA usually only makes about one mistake per 100,000 bases during the replication process, and DNA has a unique ability to detect and repair many such glitches. But a mistake left unfixed results in mutation.

Mutations that occur only in germ cells, or those that occur just after sperm and egg join, are called *de novo* mutations. *De novo* mutations often explain genetic disorders that appear suddenly, with no previous family history of the mutation. In these cases, an affected child has the mutation in every cell, and can pass it on through the family bloodline.

Some well-known genetic diseases, such as some forms of inherited colon cancer and the blood-clotting disorder hemophilia, most often originated from *de novo* mutations.

Other mutations occur later, over the course of a person's lifetime. Environmental factors often trigger such change—a tanning devotee with skin like a bronzed leather bag may wind up with a skin cell mutation and skin cancer thanks to DNA-damaging ultraviolet radiation. Other mutations can arise if an error is made while a cell and its DNA copy themselves during routine cell division. These later changes are called acquired mutations. Unless they occur in germ cells, they cannot be passed on to children. Along with UV-related skin cancer, other types of environmentally triggered cancer, such as lung cancer from smoking or thyroid cancer from excess exposure to radiation, arise from acquired mutations.

The difference in Josephine Thomas' *HFE* gene was most likely an inherited mutation. Josephine's father had symptoms of hemochromatosis, his survivors believe, and they suspect he may have died from it. Josephine's daughter, Sandra Thomas, knows that she inherited one copy of her mother's *HFE* mutation, making her a carrier.

If DNA can't always fix its mistakes, then what about doctors? Many would like to make fixes the body can't, but they don't yet have the right tools. Scientists have been trying for years to slip inside people's genes and make repairs to solve mutation-related health problems. They've made a little progress. But gene repair, or gene therapy, is extremely difficult, and its regular use remains a long way off. Gene therapy is covered more later in this book.

You don't need to wait for gene therapy breakthroughs, however, to help your DNA protect your health. If Josephine had known about her *HFE* mutation earlier, she could have protected herself in fairly simple ways. By keeping iron-rich foods out of her diet and having blood periodically withdrawn from her body to lower her iron levels, Josephine could have prevented the damage that claimed her. You, too, can make lifestyle changes and choices tailored to your particular genetic make-up. By understanding your family's genetic history and your own DNA, you can help your genes keep you healthy.

WORKING WITH YOUR GENES

As the instruction manual that built you, your genes clearly have plenty of say over your health, your body, even the very essence of who you are. But that power doesn't equal total control. Many other influences join your genes in shaping your identity and well being, and you are in charge of most of them. Your choices, your lifestyle, and the environment you live in are as influentia—and sometimes more influential—than your genes.

This balancing act, commonly framed in terms of nature versus nurture, is an important one in the era of gene science. We revisit it often throughout this book as well. But along the way, keep one solid rule of genes and health in mind: Your genes do not alone determine your fate.

Few people understand that fact better than those with an exact genomic duplicate—an identical twin. In sharing the same face with another person, identical twins know first-hand just how powerful genes can be. But they also see that power's limits, especially when it comes to health.

If genes alone determined disease, identical twins would always fall ill to the same conditions. In other words, every identical twin with diabetes would see their sibling share their illness. But identical twins, and the researchers who study them, have found that genes and illness aren't that simple. An identical twin may be at greater risk of developing diabetes if his twin is diagnosed with it first, but disease in one twin does not automatically mean disease in the other. The reasons for this largely seem to lie in what happens to each twin after their genome is formed. They may share the same genes, but life rarely deals them exactly the same hand later on.

In studies of twins and cancer, for example, identical siblings may sometimes find themselves on different paths. Two major studies of breast cancer in identical twins found that while one twin is at least three times more likely than average to develop the cancer if her sister does, she is not certain to develop the condition. While this increase in risk is important, it is also no guarantee of developing cancer. Scientists leading the studies link the different fates of some twins to external influences and personal choices, such as diet or smoking. Genes may have strong influence, but twin studies make clear that the decisions you make—what to eat, whether to smoke, whether to exercise—also influence your likelihood of illness.

Here are other key reasons why genes' influence only goes so far:

- Relatively few human illnesses are directly triggered by a single gene. Most DNA-related diseases, such as diabetes, involve many genes working together. The more genes that are involved, the better your chances that a well-functioning one can counteract one with risk-related instructions, or that you can take preventive steps to diminish a gene's affect.

- Not all genetic variations affect your health equally, due to two factors called expression and penetrance. Expression refers to the process that translates a gene's code into a physical effect. Penetrance refers to how often a variant causes an effect in the group of people who carry it. Many different factors can affect gene expression, and as a result, not all variants have equal penetrance. Hemochromatosis is a prime example of how variants can have varying effects from person to person. According to studies, at least half of all people who carry two copies of the same HFE mutation as Josephine Thomas never develop iron overload, even though they all start with the same variants.
- Instead of making you completely sick, many disease-related genes only increase your risk of getting an illness. These susceptibility genes can often be kept under control through good preventive health care. Susceptibility genes factor into many common diseases, including heart disease, asthma, breast cancer, and psoriasis.
- Genes, no matter how faulty the instructions they carry, rarely control illness on their own. Hemochromatosis, for example, worsens with a diet high in red meat, spinach, and other high-iron foods and supplements.

Those checks and balances on your genes give you plenty of opportunities to influence how they work. Through the foods you eat, the habits you keep—many of the choices you make—you have plenty of say over how your genes run your body. Here are just a few examples. Many more are covered in greater detail throughout this book.

- Make a record of illnesses that are common among your relatives. This family medical history often reveals inherited diseases and health risks, pointing you and your doctors to preventive care that protects you. To learn more about creating a family medical history, see Chapter 2.
- Good nutrition helps you keep your genes healthy and functioning properly. A healthful diet can also counterbalance genetic risk. People who inherit an increased risk for diabetes, for example, can ward off the condition and its complications by avoiding excess starches, sugar, and fat. Genes and nutrition are discussed more in Chapter 5.
- Avoid habits known to trigger acquired mutations. As mentioned earlier, common activities such as smoking and too much sun exposure often lead to dangerous cancer-causing mutations. To find out more about acquired mutations and cancer, see Chapter 6.

No outside influence can strip your genome of its risks entirely. But knowing your genes' quirks and inclinations can give you important insights into your instruction manual. Genomic knowledge can guide you to steps that will help your genes build better health.

YOUR GENES: SPECIAL CONSIDERATIONS

Throughout the rest of this book, we talk in more detail about individual genes, certain illnesses, and what you can do about them. Before getting that specific, though, it's worth pointing out a few more gene essentials especially important for men, women, and different ethnic groups.

X and Y: The Male-Female Divide

A little earlier, we talked about the different sets of sex chromosomes in men and women. Men carry an unmatched set—XY. For women, it's an XX.

The Y chromosome, consisting of roughly 80 genes, focuses on

Diagnosis Uncovers Family "Secret"

Already the mother of a little girl, Erin was thrilled to deliver a son. Her sister had a boy a year earlier, so Michael was the second grandson. Both boys were a joy to their grandparents, who had three daughters, but no sons.

Michael was three when they attended their first family reunion. The whole family was excited to see each other, as well as to hike to parts of the Grand Canyon. By day three, both mothers noticed that the boys struggled with the hikes. However, they were troupers, and with a minimum amount of whining, the boys kept up with the older sisters.

Back home, Erin was thrilled to learn that she was pregnant again; she and her husband Brian had wanted three children. During the pregnancy, Erin spent time preparing the kids for a new sister or brother. And she also began to worry about Michael's clumsiness—was he acting out because he would not receive as much attention? An orthopedist declared that he was fine. However, he walked on his tiptoes a lot, something his sister never did.

That Labor Day, Erin was watching the Muscular Dystrophy Telethon. One of the little boys on the program moved exactly like Michael! With her heart in her throat, she called her pediatrician for an appointment. She wanted to know if her son had a problem—and she wasn't leaving the office until she had an answer.

She got one. At age four, Michael was diagnosed with Duchenne Muscular Dystrophy (DMD), a progressive disease that causes contractures of the muscles around the joints, especially in the pelvis, upper arms, and upper legs. This results in a loss of mobility, and most boys with DMD are unable to walk by the time they reach their mid teens.

Erin was devastated and could not quit crying for days. What was going to happen to Michael? What if the child she was carrying was also affected? She was so anxious that her doctor sent her for a genetic consultation. Prior to the visit, Erin provided information about Michael's diagnosis as well as health information about other family members. While collecting the information, Erin learned for the first shaping male characteristics. X, by contrast, is busy doing a lot more! With more than 1,000 genes, X not only shapes female traits but also carries the instructions for many other parts of the body. Instructions for everything from helping your blood clot to enabling you to see red and green sit on your X chromosome.

With their two Xs, women carry a double set of all those important instructions. They have a backup if something goes wrong. Men have just one set. That difference creates some important health differences. Here's how that happens.

If You're a Man . . .

With only one set of X instructions in their bodies, men have no backup if one of their X-related instructions carries a risk-related difference. These faulty genes start giving orders in their bodies, as they are the only version of those orders to follow.

time that her mother had a brother who died when he was 14. The family had never spoken about it.

After getting family member information and reviewing the doctor's evaluation of DMD, the genetic counselor shared with Erin and her husband that this condition is inherited in an X-linked manner. The uncle she never knew was a clue that the genetic alteration that caused DMD in her family likely began in an earlier generation.

There was much to discuss: Michael; the current pregnancy; and other family members. Mostly, it would take time to understand Michael's condition and what they could do to minimize problems. Their most immediate concern was the current pregnancy, and the genetic counselor explained that a daughter would be unaffected, but if they had a son, he would have a 50% chance of having DMD. An ultrasound showed that the baby was most likely a girl, and this was later confirmed by chromosome analysis. Last, and most difficult, Erin called her sister with the news—the boys were too similar, with large calf muscles and difficulty running, for Erin's nephew to not also be affected. She encouraged her sister to go to their pediatrician. About a month later, Erin was again heartbroken, but not surprised, to learn that her nephew had DMD.

Two years later, the family has learned much about DMD, participated in summer camps, and encouraged Michael to participate as actively as he is able. There are two young men in the support group who are in their early 20s and an inspiration that Michael's "normal" is just different now.

Bottom Line: As a genetic counselor, I encourage parents to be aware and persistent when their child's differences seem problematic. Michael's big calves and clumsiness were clues to his diagnosis. In addition, encouraging family communication about health history is so important. Erin's uncle was an important piece to this story. She learned from this "family secret" how important it is that her daughters be informed of their potential carrier status when they are old enough to understand.

This explains why certain X-linked genetic problems appear much more often in men than in women. Hemophilia, a blood-clotting disorder, occurs far more often in men. The same goes for red-green color blindness. Many other conditions, including some forms of mental retardation and Duchenne Muscular Dystrophy, also appear more often in men, simply because their related genes sit on the X chromosome. Such conditions are called sex-linked disorders, as they sit on a sex-related chromosome.

If you are a man with a sex-linked disorder, you pass your affected gene on to any daughters you may have through your X chromosome. When they inherit your gene, they become carriers, but will not usually develop illness from just one copy of the gene. You can help them keep their children healthier by having your family work with genetic specialists skilled at detecting and treating sex-linked disorders. These specialists are covered in Chapter 2.

If You're a Woman . . .

With two Xs, women rarely develop sex-linked disorders. One of their Xs may carry risk-related instructions, but there is a good chance their other X will carry correct instructions and work as the dominant gene. Women who are carriers of a faulty gene on X can pass this gene on to their children, but they don't often get sick themselves.

If you are a woman who carries a sex-linked disorder, you can pass your affected gene on to daughters or sons. If your children inherit your affected gene, your sons may become sick from it, while your daughters will become carriers. If you carry a sex-linked disorder, seek help from genetic specialists skilled at detecting and treating such conditions. These specialists are covered in Chapter 2.

Ethnic Groups

As we discussed earlier, some small DNA changes, such as polymorphisms and SNP's, have noticeable effects. Many of the external differences between groups of people—the variations in skin color, stature, or eye shape that society calls ethnicity or race—arise from these small DNA variations.

Gene scientists have also discovered that differences between population groups aren't limited to what we can see. Some gene-related diseases, such as hemochromatosis, appear more often in some populations than others. People of Irish, Scottish, or English heritage, such as Josephine Thomas, carry the hemochromatosis mutation at much higher rates than people from most other parts of the world. Africans and people of African heritage suffer from sickle-cell anemia, a genetic blood disorder, more often than other groups. These health differences also arise from polymorphisms.

An important global research effort is using DNA samples from groups around the world to better understand how polymorphisms cluster in certain populations and how they affect health. Called the International HapMap Project, (Hap, short for haplotype, is gene-speak for a set of

Putting Differences to Good Use

Scientists who published the first map of the human genome in 2001 used the announcement to present their case that there is no genetic basis for the concept of race.

"Any two humans on this planet are more than 99.9 percent identical at the molecular level. Racial and ethnic differences are all indeed only skin deep," said Eric Lander, then director of one of the major labs that contributed to the project.

As we all know, though, discussions of race are rarely that straightforward. The concepts of race, ethnicity, and racial differences are deeply ingrained in human culture. As much as gene scientists like to say that there is no genetic basis for race, they also realize they can't ignore the concept's social role.

That acknowledgment has helped shape important international research projects that look at tiny DNA differences between population groups. As we mentioned in this chapter, these small differences sometimes have important effects on health, causing certain illnesses—or resistance to those illnesses—to cluster in certain populations. This research is helping to find disease risks in certain groups, and may also eventually drive targeted preventions and treatments.

We look more closely at these population-specific conditions and research projects throughout this book. Scientists may be studying these population differences, but they ultimately hope their work serves a universal goal—that of keeping more of us in better health.

closely linked alleles), the program is helping medical experts link polymorphisms to common diseases such as asthma and heart disease.

Does all this add up to big gene differences between races? Most scientists quickly say, "No." The differences between people we describe as race are actually small, and say far more about history, geography, and health than they do other aspects of human life. While the concept of race has strong social meaning, numerous scientific studies have determined that there are no genes that spell it out. There is no single gene, for example, that makes someone white, black, or Latino.

In fact, two people who appear to be of the same race may actually have very few significant gene factors in common. This is especially true for those of mixed heritage. Two individuals lumped together as African-American, for example, may be of mixed African, European, and Native American ancestry, and have DNA far more similar to one of those groups than they do to each other.

Human history appears to be the force that has caused some polymorphisms and SNPs to cluster in different population groups. After people slowly spread across the globe—moving from Africa to Asia and Europe, or later from Asia to the Americas—distance kept groups separate for thousands of years. Groups of people could swap genes in relative isolation, slowly developing DNA that reflected their environment. We may live in a global melting pot now, but those patterns of rapid human migration and mixing are relatively recent.

Telling Your Own Gene Story

Josephine Thomas discovered her *HFE* mutation near the end of her life. She had started treatment, having blood drawn regularly to lower her iron count, but it was too late. Her liver, badly damaged from years of high iron, was succumbing to cancer.

But Josephine wanted her illness to mean something beyond family tragedy. She and her daughter Sandra started sharing the family's story. They spread the word about hemochromatosis, especially among people of Irish, Scottish, or English descent who might be at higher risk. Josephine wrote articles and appeared on television, urging others to seek gene testing. Sandra founded the American Hemochromatosis Society, which provides information on testing, symptoms, and treatment. She openly discusses her own status as an *HFE* mutation carrier.

"It was my mother's dying wish that everyone be tested for hemochromatosis," Sandra said.

Talking about genes and illness is a powerful way to spread the word about everyone's new options in gene-related health care. Sharing your story might help others learn about new treatments, or reduce the feelings of isolation that gene concerns sometimes bring. Not everyone is comfortable with taking their genes public, and no one will fault you for guarding your privacy. But today's forms of communication, especially online media, give all of us powerful options for sharing our stories. If you are thinking about making your story part of the growing public discussion on genes and health, gene experts suggest considering these issues:

- Make sure you think through the implications of making your genomic information public. Telling your story to a group of strangers online is one thing. Would you be comfortable having that same story shared with your co-workers or neighbors? For more information on privacy issues, see Chapter 8.
- Talk with your family about your decision. Your genes are connected to theirs. If your relatives' gene information will also be shared in some way, do they agree with your choice? For more information on talking with your family, see Chapter 2.
- See how sharing your information might benefit you. Some people with particular health conditions, for example, find value in sharing detailed accounts of their health with others online, swapping experiences, and treatment suggestions. Others prefer a doctor's advice to that of strangers, and would rather not discuss personal health issues in public. To find some examples of these types of gene- and health-related forums, please see the Resources section at the end of this book.

We look more closely at specific ethnic health issues throughout this book, but to give a sense of how genes play out in certain populations, here are some broad ways genes affect the health of some groups:

African-Americans and Africans

In addition to sickle-cell anemia, African-Americans also develop many forms of heart disease and some cancers, such as prostate cancer, at higher rates than other groups in the United States. While many factors beside genes affect heart health and cancer, scientists suspect gene variations influence how some African-Americans develop these conditions.

Asian-Americans and Asians

Descendants of populations from southeast and south Asia carry higher rates of thalassemia, a group of blood disorders that affect the blood's ability to carry oxygen.

Caucasians

Jews of European descent are at higher risk for a range of genetic illnesses, including the childhood neurological disease Tay-Sachs and some forms of breast cancer. In addition to hemochromatosis, people of northern European descent are also at higher risk for cystic fibrosis, a glandular disorder that can affect breathing, digestion, and reproduction.

Latinos

Rates of diabetes are higher than the norm among Latinos in the United States. While many diet and lifestyle factors affect diabetes, scientists suspect some Latinos may also have more genetic risk.

Native Americans

Some Native American tribes have the highest known rates of diabetes in the world. Again, diet and lifestyle are likely contributors, but some scientists say some tribes show susceptibility genes that drive up their diabetic risk.

If you're concerned about genetic risks linked to your ethnic background, you can start protecting your health by learning what genetic illnesses are most common among people in your ethnic group. Some of these illnesses and their ethnic links are covered in later chapters. If you can't find information in the book about a health issue of interest to you, go to the Resources section, which lists ways to find additional information.

You can find the most thorough information by talking to your doctor or a specialist in genetic conditions. Some of these types of experts are introduced in Chapter 2.

FREQUENTLY ASKED QUESTIONS ABOUT GENES AND HOW THEY WORK

Q. My neighbor has a son with Down syndrome, which she says comes from a problem with too many chromosomes. Is that possible?

A. Down syndrome, a developmental disorder, is one of several conditions arising from an extra chromosome in a person's genome. These extra chromosomes usually appear when a genetic error produces them in sex cells. People with Down syndrome, for example, have three copies of Chromosome 21 instead of the normal two. For more details on Down syndrome and other chromosome conditions, turn to Chapter 4.

Q. If children inherit their parents' genes, why do they sometimes look so different from them? Some kids have really different features from their parents. In our family, my daughter looks nothing like me or my wife, but she does look like my wife's mother.

A. The tricks genes play as they form sex cells and make babies often mean that families see some gene-related surprises in their newest members. Remember that your germ cells shuffle bits of your DNA as they form your sperm or eggs. A sex cell can also shuffle that DNA some more as it combines with another to start making a baby. This process, called recombination, leads to a new genome a little different from its parent genomes.

In forming sex cells, germ cells also have the option of working with all your DNA, not just the DNA that gave you your appearance. For example, your wife got the genes related to appearance from both her mother and her father. Her father's genes may have sculpted her outward features, but her mother's genes are still in her genome, available to be passed on in sex cells. Appearance-related genes from your wife's mother may have wound up in one of your wife's eggs and been passed on to your daughter. That's how your daughter can look like Grandma, even if your wife doesn't.

Q. My father had hemochromatosis, and I just found out I'm a carrier. Will I get sick from iron overload?

A. Since carriers have only one copy of a risk-related gene, they often don't get sick from it, although they can still pass the gene on to their children. In a few cases, however, carriers may experience some health effects from their single copy of a mutation. Hemochromatosis is one such instance—carriers may have slightly higher iron levels than normal, for example. If you are a hemochromatosis carrier, you can take preventive steps to detect elevated iron levels and ward off problems, so talk with your doctor or a genetic specialist.

Q. If I find out I have genetic mutation, does that automatically mean I'm going to get sick?

A. No. A mutation is only a change in a gene. It can be a helpful change, a harmful change, or completely neutral. Most mutations are not harmful. If you do have a risk-related mutation, you can sometimes take important steps to lower your risk. Many of these preventive measures are covered throughout this book.

Q. My father is Chinese and my mother is Caucasian, with ancestors from Germany. My best friend is also of mixed heritage. She is a Latina from Puerto Rico, and her ancestors come from Africa,

Europe, and the Caribbean. How do ethnic links to genetic disease affect mixed race people?

A. People of mixed race have gene diversity working to their advantage. If a disease-linked mutation that clusters in a particular ethnic group runs on one side of their family, it is far less likely to run on the other. For example, people of northern European descent, such as your mother, are at higher risk for carrying the most common mutation for cystic fibrosis. But people from Asia, such as your father, are at lower risk. If you had inherited the cystic fibrosis mutation from your mother, your father's gene would likely counteract it.

If you are considering some type of genetic evaluation, your diversity brings both benefits and risks. Health care providers may offer you a broader range of gene tests, covering issues relevant to all your ancestral ethnicities. But at the same time, not all gene tests are currently sensitive enough to detect risk-related genes in some ethnic groups. For more information on this testing dilemma, see Chapter 4.

KEEP IN MIND

As you start using basic gene-speak to understand your genes and help them keep you healthy, here are some key points to remember:

- Your genes begin with bases, genetic letters that spell out all the words, paragraphs, and chapters of the instruction manual that built your body. Sometimes, having just one different base in a key place can have an important effect on your health.
- Your genes make more of themselves, and copy themselves to renew your body.
- Your genome also makes slightly different copies of itself to create your children.
- Changes in your DNA are called mutations, and most of them aren't harmful. Some mutations can be as small as a single letter change, a mutation called an SNP.
- Genes have a lot of say when it comes to your body, your identity, and your health. But outside factors, such as your diet and your habits, also have plenty of influence over your well-being. Your health isn't all in your DNA—much of it rests in your hands.

Now that you understand the essentials of how your genes work, you're ready to begin creating a tool for yourself and your family that can help point the way to better health—your personal genomic guidebook.

CHAPTER TWO

READING YOUR GENETIC OPERATING INSTRUCTIONS

Thanks to genetic screening, Kevin Lewis learned that a poor showing on a test could actually be a lifesaver.

In the mid-1990s, with gene science just starting to make big moves into medical care, Kevin and his family got a chance to peer inside their DNA. Many of Kevin's relatives, including his dad and grandmother, had suffered from colon cancer and other malignancies. A team of scientists studying links between genes and colon cancer learned of the family's history and offered them a test to see if a heightened risk of cancer ran in the family bloodline.

Kevin signed up. When his results arrived, he found himself facing equal doses of fear and hope. "DNA sequencing analysis of...the *MSH2* gene indicates that the mutation at IVS11-1(G>A) previously detected in this family is present," the results read. "Genetic counseling is recommended."

Kevin's *MSH2* gene mutation on Chromosome 2 is linked to Lynch syndrome, after Dr. Henry Lynch, who initially described this type of hereditary colon cancer. In addition to colon cancer, this mutation also increases the risk of stomach, liver, and other cancers, often at a young age.

Kevin, now in his 40s, points out that his ominous test result was anything but a failure. Instead, he says, the knowledge that he carries this mutation has infused his life with new energy and power. He started undergoing yearly colon cancer screenings, which caught several pre-cancerous polyps early so they could be removed. He co-founded the Colon Cancer Alliance, a patient support and advocacy group, and speaks often about the need for improved colon cancer screening. He went from wondering about his cancer risk to reducing it. He started using the information in his genes to protect himself and help others.

"I represent future colorectal cancer patients in a unique and special way," Kevin says. "The problem is that the special knowledge that my family has is extremely rare. Most families do not have this information. We were part of a special genome study. This study gave me a special lease on my life, and I will do everything in my power to make sure that the medical community continues to learn how to screen, prevent, and treat this dreaded disease."

In turning his DNA from a mystery into useful medical information, Kevin shows just how deeply genomic tests can remake health. New advances, arriving at a rapid clip, are allowing more of us to bring our genetic information into our plans for a healthier future. You can now learn more about your DNA than ever before and find a growing group of doctors and genetic counselors to help you make the most of that information. With each new opportunity to read your genomic instruction manual, your health care will take a more personal turn.

This shift to personalized medicine comes in many forms. Your doctor may tell you about a promising prescription drug designed to work well with certain varieties of genes. You may learn of a new DNA test that you can obtain through your doctor, or select for yourself online. Important news that connects your genes to your health makes the pages of newspapers, magazines, and medical journals every week. Split into so many pieces, the magnitude of this genomic shift can sometimes be hard to absorb. But put together, the elements of personalized medicine are remaking your options for better health. Here are key pieces in the personalized medical kit you can now assemble:

- A detailed family medical history, drafted by hand or computer. A family medical history reveals what conditions run in your bloodline, pointing out health risks you may face. Federal health officials now encourage every American to create a family medical history, and provide the tools to do so.
- Genetic testing to reveal your inherited risk for diseases such as breast cancer, colon cancer, or celiac disease. Some of these tests, such as those that look specifically at gene mutations related to breast or colon cancer risk, are scientifically proven and well established. Others, such as tests that scan your genome for DNA related to multiple conditions at once or that claim to detect your risk of developing Alzheimer's disease, are newer and less proven. A few, such as genetic tests that claim to gauge your genetic need for a particular type of vitamin, have earned widespread scientific skepticism. You'll encounter this variety—and controversy—often as you start bringing your DNA into your health plans, and you'll need to consider your options carefully.
- Genetic testing that diagnoses disease. Doctors usually use these tests, generally the oldest in the genomic medical kit, to confirm a diagnosis of genetic illnesses such as the neurological disorder Huntington's disease or the pediatric condition called Fragile X.

You can also turn to such tests to spot chromosomal or gene abnormalities in pregnancy, or to look for risk-related genes in your relatives if someone in the family has a confirmed genetic illness.

- Drugs that match DNA features in some people. This blend of drugs and gene science, known as pharmacogenomics, is still in its infancy, but it is developing quickly. In some cancer cases, for example, analysis of a cancer cell's particular DNA-based traits reveal whether certain tumor-fighting drugs offer improved prospects for stopping the cancer. Many gene scientists predict that this blend of an individual's genes and medicines will soon move beyond cancer, becoming a routine part of prescribing many medicines. In their plans for the future, you'll eventually be able to select drugs tailored to your genes.
- Genetic testing to establish a person's identity, including paternity testing and lineage testing to reveal ethnic ancestry. While such tests don't fall neatly into the medical realm, they may have health implications, as a better understanding of a person's ancestry may reveal new health insights.
- Gene banking, in which DNA from thousands or millions of people is stored and used for research and medical experimentation. Federal agencies, university research centers, and health care organizations are setting up these DNA warehouses, offering the promise of medical breakthroughs. But the collecting of all that genetic data also raises questions about how it will be used and protected.

You may be thinking this genomic system, while ambitious, sounds somewhat remote. How much will your DNA really be used to determine the course of your health care anytime soon? The answer is that personalized medicine is already here. One piece of your genomic medical kit, your family medical history, is as close as a computer keyboard or pad of paper. Other pieces, such as genetic tests for conditions or risk of disease, are available from genetic specialists, your family doctor, and even over the Internet. More and more are expected to be available before long. Dr. Francis Collins, the first director of the federal Human Genome Research Institute, predicts the United States will need just 25 years or so to reach a fully DNA-based system of health care.

By 2020, Collins says, gene-based designer drugs will probably be available for conditions such as diabetes, Alzheimer's disease, and high blood pressure. Cancer treatment will expand in its ability to kill or limit tumors by targeting their DNA fingerprints. Your genetic information will be a routine part of prescribing your medicines, and genomic knowledge will transform the entire system of diagnosing and treating mental illness.

And by the year 2030, Collins predicts, comprehensive, genomics-based health care will become the norm, with individualized preventive medicine and early detection of illnesses long before symptoms arise. Gene therapy, treatments that involve altering your genome itself, will be available for many diseases.

As you start bringing your genetic information into your personal health plans, though, it's important to know that genomic care still has its limits. Genomic insights will often provide insight into your risk of developing a particular health condition, rather than a certainty that it will or will not occur. Other limits arise from the imbalance between DNA-based diagnosis and actual treatment. The ability to diagnose some DNA-related conditions far outpaces our ability to treat them. This doesn't leave you without options for treating gene-related conditions. But it does mean that those treatments may not match the sophistication of the screening that detected your problem in the first place. Kevin Lewis, for example, took advantage of a sophisticated gene test to detect his colon cancer risk. But when that risk became apparent, the procedures available to him—regular screenings and the surgical removal of potentially cancerous polyps—were no different from those offered to other patients undergoing colon screening.

You'll also have costs to consider. Genome scans, which examine your DNA for multiple SNPs related to many different conditions, usually cost at least several hundred dollars and are typically not covered by insurance policies. Gene tests for single conditions range from hundreds to thousands of dollars. If you have health insurance, and your doctor and insurance company approve your genomic testing or care, most of your costs will be covered. But if you don't have insurance, or your policy is limited, you may face higher out-of-pocket costs. If you choose to avoid involving your insurer and pay for your tests or care yourself, you'll have to cover the entire bill.

These issues arise in many different aspects of genomic care, and we address them often in this book. You'll also receive invaluable guidance from genomic care providers who can help you unlock the health information carried in your DNA.

STEP 1: CHOOSE A GENETIC HEALTH PROVIDER

As genomic innovations unfold, you may already be lucky enough to have a family doctor well versed in the basics of genomic care. But not all family physicians are trained in genomic medicine—many doctors have as hard a time keeping up with all the latest developments as the rest of us. That often means you'll be sent to specialized caregivers if you're seeking genetic help. Some of these specialists, called genetic counselors, aren't found in other fields of medicine. Others, such as specialized doctors and nurses, will be more familiar to you.

Your Family Doctor

As your primary caregiver, your regular doctor is often your first stop in seeking gene-related care. Some front-line physicians are working quickly to incorporate genomics into their medical practice, taking advantage of new training that blends gene science into everyday medicine. If your doctor is one of these pioneers, she is also likely comfortable discussing simpler family history concerns, genetic testing, or treatment options with you. She may, however, refer you to a specialist for more complex questions.

If your care starts with your family physician, ask about your doctor's experience with genomic medicine. Some primary care doctors, for example, seek training from groups such as the National Coalition for Health Professional Education in Genetics (NCHPEG). This group, made up of gene experts, offers training in genomic medicine to primary care doctors, nurses, and physician assistants. NCHPEG's training includes everything from the basics of gene science to helping doctors understand how genomic concerns affect different ethnic groups. If your physician has not yet had the opportunity to participate in further genomic training, you may want to consider asking for a referral to a genetic or genomic specialist. Some of these specialists also accept self-referrals.

Once you have sought specialty care, here are some of the gene experts you'll likely encounter.

Genetic Counselors

These professionals fill a unique role in genomic care. Genetic counselors are not doctors, and they cannot provide treatment themselves. But they are a powerful health-care team member in your effort to understand your genes and keep yourself healthy. You'll usually be sent to one if you have gene-related questions that your regular doctor isn't comfortable answering, or if you select genetic testing or other gene-related care.

Think of genetic counselors as your personal guide to your genetic health care options. They offer understanding of both DNA science and the real-life complexities of your genetic choices. Genetic counselors can help you:

- Assess your risk of a genetic disorder by helping you research your family history and medical records.
- Weigh your medical, social, and ethical decisions surrounding your genetic tests.

Genomic Training for Ethnic-Specific Conditions

The National Coalition for Health Professional Education in Genetics trains medical caregivers in more than just gene science. They also include information specific to ethnic minorities, coaching doctors and nurses on genomic issues relevant to African-Americans, Latinos, and other ethnic groups. If you're a member of an ethnic minority, ask your caregivers if they're familiar, either through training or caring for other patients, with gene issues specific to your ethnic community.

- Make a decision about testing by providing information and emotional support.
- Interpret the results of your genetic tests and medical data.
- Find further counseling and support services should you need them.
- Work with your doctors, hospital, or other health-care providers.
- Understand possible treatments or preventive measures.

Expectant parents considering a genetic test before their baby is born, for example, usually meet with a genetic counselor to learn about the test and how it works. The counselor will explain the test's benefits and limitations, and help the couple interpret test results. But the counselor will also go beyond the mechanics of the test, helping them sort through the complex issues surrounding it. Will insurance cover it? What do their personal beliefs say about taking the test or acting on its results? Is the test right for them, not just medically, but emotionally?

When you meet with a genetic counselor, your session will be tailored to your individual situation. But counselors say the following features will likely be a part of your visit:

- Going over your medical history and genetic care to date in detail. While some of this information may be contained in records the genetic counselor reviews beforehand, a counselor will likely seek more information. Counselors are also better informed on genomics than most health-care practitioners, and they may think to ask questions others would miss.
- Spending a good part of the visit talking about your situation, questions, and needs. Unlike many doctors, who are used to dispensing treatments and advice in quick appointments, counselors hold detailed conversations with patients and families to uncover as many useful gene-related details as possible. They also usually reserve a substantial part of the visit for patient questions.
- Being presented with choices rather than instructions. Counselors focus on helping patients make their own personal decisions that are right for them. A counselor will help you understand your options, benefits, and risks in the realm of genomic care.
- Talking about a wide range of topics. Your genes touch every aspect of your life, and conversations with a genetic counselor usually go far beyond the mechanics of medicine. Counselors help patients with everything from privacy issues and health insurance to the emotional effects of genetic test results. And because genetics is about families, the discussion will often include the impact of the result on your family members, as well.

Medical Geneticists

Medical geneticists are doctors who specialize in genetic disease. The vast majority are also pediatricians who work primarily with birth defects or childhood diseases. Others work with a wide variety of conditions. Visiting these specialists usually requires a referral from your regular doctor.

Medical geneticists work closely with genetic counselors to offer a thorough range of care to their patients. As with any type of doctor, personality and "bedside manner" have a lot to say about your relationship with a medical geneticist. Some talk with their patients in detail, providing in-depth answers and emotional support. Others stick to the business of medicine, and leave the longer conversation to your genetic counselor.

Genetic Nurses

Genetic nurses are licensed professional nurses with special training in genetics. Some offer care similar to that of genetic counselors, helping patients and families with risk assessment for genetic disease. They also offer specialized care to patients with genetic illness, helping administer medicines and other types of treatment required to manage a genetic medical condition.

How to Find a Genomic Specialist

When your doctor refers you to a genetic specialist, that referral usually connects you to a network of counselors and medical geneticists that your doctor respects and works with often. But in some cases, you may find yourself looking for a specialist on your own. If you have insurance that doesn't require your doctor's approval for specialty care, for example, you can seek specialty care as you like. You may feel that you need genomic help more quickly than your regular doctor can provide it, perhaps because a relative has received genetic testing results that raise questions for your own health.

If you're looking for a specialist on your own, here are some places to start, along with some ways to make sure you'll be getting quality care.

If you're looking for a medical geneticist, a good place to start is the American College of Medical Genetics. This group represents doctors who specialize in genomic care, working to advance the use of medical genetics and use of genomics to improve public health. It provides services to help you find medical geneticists in your area at www.acmg.net. Most medical geneticists carry credentials that show they've received specialty training. Most, for example, are certified by the American Board of Medical Genetics. One you find a specialist, ask your doctor if he has undergone any special training or certification. If you have questions about your doctor's overall practice record, contact your state medical board to see if your doctor is licensed, and if his record shows any violations or disciplinary actions. If you're looking for a genetic counselor, a great place to start is the National Society of Genetic Counselors. This professional group represents counselors all over the country, and the group's website, www.nsgc.org, includes features that let you search for a counselor by region, by name, or by specialty.

Genetic counselors have advanced degrees in genetic counseling and are usually certified by the American Board of Genetic Counseling. Many states are now passing laws regarding licensure for genetic counselors, and those laws already exist in Illinois, Massachusetts, Oklahoma, and Utah. Ask your genetic counselor about her training and professional affiliations.

Seeking Your Own DNA Analysis

Some people, however, aren't waiting to get tested through an established medical provider, opting instead for DNA testing through an organization that allows the public to order DNA analysis directly.

In this realm, you can choose to bypass doctors and insurers by signing up for a test through a private company or publicly funded research project. In commercial testing services, you can usually, for a fee, select either a specific test or select from a range of DNA tests, submit a DNA sample, and review your DNA information yourself. Some of these services include genetic counseling, while others do not. Hundreds of companies now sell some form of DNA analysis online, covering everything from paternity testing to gene scans that assess your risk for multiple health conditions at once. At least one publicly funded genetic analysis effort, the Coriell Personalized Medicine Collaborative, offers DNA testing for free as part of a research project. If you choose to participate, their research priorities and guidelines will define how your genetic information is analyzed.

These self-driven approaches hold appeal for people concerned about speed and privacy. You don't have to wait for a doctor's visit or genetic counseling appointment. If you sign up with a commercial company, you may choose the tests that interest you, without a doctor's approval. The results go directly to you, without entering your medical record.

But this route to DNA testing, often called direct-to-consumer testing, remains one of the most debated areas in genomic medicine. Many of the companies offering direct-to-consumer tests strive to offer ethical, reliable genomic care. But some of these companies are not subject to the same rules or codes of conduct you'll find in a regular doctor's office. Nor do some of them offer the same level of guidance you'd receive from a qualified genetic counselor. If you're interested in trying direct-to-consumer DNA tests, here are a few issues to consider:

- Federal laws do not ensure the validity of most genetic tests, including those offered to direct-to-consumer companies. Doctors and genetic counselors who routinely handle hundreds or thousands of tests a year know how to watch for quality and spot problems. But individual consumers have few ways to make sure they are getting quality testing from a direct-to-consumer company. In 2006, federal lawmakers began pushing for greater regulation of direct-to-consumer tests.
- Some direct-to-consumer tests may be of little actual value, analyzing DNA with unclear connections to disease. Some tests, for

◢ RED FLAG!

At-Home Gene Tests: What to Watch For

In a warning to consumers in mid-2006, the Federal Trade Commission issued the following guidelines for people considering direct-to-consumer genetic tests:

- Talk to your doctor or health-care practitioner about whether genetic testing might provide useful information about your health, and if so, which test would be best. Make sure you understand the benefits and limits of any test before you buy it—or take it.
- Ask your doctor or a genetic counselor to help you understand your test results. Many companies that sell at-home genetic tests do not interpret the results for you.
- Discuss the results of your test with your doctor or health-care practitioner before making any dietary or other health-related decisions following the test. Genetic test results can be complex and serious. You don't want to make any decisions based on incomplete, inaccurate, or misunderstood information.
- Protect your privacy. Some direct-to-consumer test companies may post patient test results online. If the website is not secure, your information may be seen by others. Before you do business with any company online, check the privacy policy to see how they may use your personal information, and whether they share customer information with marketers or other third parties.
- While most other home-use medical tests undergo FDA review to provide a reasonable assurance of their safety and effectiveness, no at-home genetic tests have been reviewed by the FDA, and the FDA has not evaluated the accuracy of their claims.

In short, federal officials, along with gene experts, say you need to be extra well-informed if you're going to use a direct-to-consumer genetic test. Ask detailed questions before paying any money to such a company, and don't act on the results of any such test before talking with your doctor.

example, offer to look for DNA related to obesity, but do not clearly state that most links between obesity and the DNA being tested are tenuous, or that the DNA in question only has limited power over your weight.

- Some testing companies do not offer the service of genetic counselors, leaving patients to interpret complex results themselves. This is especially problematic when tests only indicate risk, rather than providing a clear "Yes" or "No" answer. If you undergo a direct-to-consumer test that reveals your risk of cancer is 40 percent higher than normal, what does that number really mean? What should you do? Some companies do not provide genetic experts to help you answer such questions.
- These tests are usually expensive, often costing hundreds or thousands of dollars, and most insurance companies do not cover the

cost, if you choose to involve your insurer at all. Many people choosing these tests pay the costs out of their own pockets.

- Since almost all these companies only offer testing, not medical care, any medically important results will still mean seeking out a doctor's help. You often won't be able to rely on these tests to answer most of your medical questions.

To address these concerns, genetic counselors offer the following suggestions:

- Before you hand over any money to a direct-to-consumer testing company, ask the company what its test means. Will it show if you have a mutation that causes disease? Will it show if you have increased susceptibility or risk?
- Does the company offer any data or expertise that helps you know if your results mean that you'll get sick from any of the genetic insights the test uncovers? If not, can the company help you find that information?
- The National Society of Genetic Counselors recommends that most genetic test results be given face to face, by a knowledgeable medical professional who has an established relationship with the patient. Many direct-to-consumer companies do not offer this level of counseling. Ask the company what, if any, genetic counseling they offer. If they do offer some form of counseling, ask what kind of training and credentials the counselors carry.
- Consider how you'll use your test results in the future. If your test results point to an increased risk of illness or a medical problem, you should share your genetic information with your doctors so that you receive appropriate care. But you might also someday be asked to disclose your information to some types of insurers, such as those that provide disability or long-term care coverage. These types of insurers currently have fewer legal restrictions against using your genetic information in making their insurance decisions. (For more information on insurance concerns, see Chapter 8.)

As you choose your own path to understanding the health information your DNA holds, you'll be able to rely on a wide range of tools. Some are surprisingly simple. Others rely on highly specialized labs and complex DNA analysis.

To get started, your entry into personalized medicine requires nothing more high-tech than pencil and paper and a few conversations with your relatives.

STEP 2: CREATE YOUR FAMILY MEDICAL HISTORY

Your family medical history is one of your most powerful tools for assessing your risk of genetic conditions. Family history is most easily compiled and studied by creating a family history chart, also known as a family pedigree. Genetic counselors routinely draw up such family trees for their patients. The documents closely resemble family trees created to trace genealogy, with one notable addition. These family trees also track the appearance of diseases or health problems alongside births, deaths, and marriages.

Documenting your family's medical history can reveal tendencies to develop certain types of cancers, for example, or early heart disease. Once these health patterns become apparent, you and your doctor can use them to help diagnose medical problems, develop plans for disease prevention, identify other family members who may also need medical attention, and gauge the risk of passing these conditions on to your children.

While genetic counselors routinely draw up family medical histories as part of their work with patients, you don't need expert help to get started. Free guidelines and tools are now widely available to help families create their own medical histories. One place you can start is the Web site for "My Family Health Portrait," an Internet-based kit developed by the U.S. Surgeon General's office. At www.hhs.gov/familyhistory/, you'll find software that lets you create your family medical history online or on your own computer. You can also download and print a paper version to develop by hand. The Surgeon General's kit formally tracks common health conditions—heart disease, stroke, diabetes, colon cancer, breast cancer, and ovarian cancer—and includes room for others. The Surgeon General's office says any use of their family history tools remains private.

If you prefer to draft your family history on paper, the National Society of Genetic Counselors offers these suggestions:

One way to record a family history is by drawing a family tree called a pedigree. A pedigree looks very much like a traditional family tree. You can also create and keep a written list of your family information without drawing a pedigree. You'll find an example of a pedigree on page 45.

Whether or not you draw a formal pedigree, begin by writing down the medical and health information on:

• Yourself	• Your children
• Your brothers and sisters	• Your parents

Then add a generation at a time. Include:

• Nieces and nephews	• Grandparents
• Aunts and uncles	• Cousins

For each relative, try to write down as many of these items as possible:

Age or date of birth (and, for all family members who have passed on, age at death and cause of death). When the information is unavailable, write down your best guess (for example, 40s). If you are noting the ages, include the date that you collected the information.

Medical problems, noting the ages at which the conditions occurred. Did Uncle Pete have his heart attack at age 42 or age 88? Did your mother develop diabetes in childhood or as an adult? Include conditions such as:

- Cancer
- Diabetes
- Mental illness
- Stroke
- Alcoholism

- Heart disease
- Asthma
- High blood pressure
- Kidney disease
- Learning problems, mental retardation.

- Birth defects such as spina bifida, cleft lip, heart defects, others.
- Vision loss/hearing loss at a young age (record the age it began).

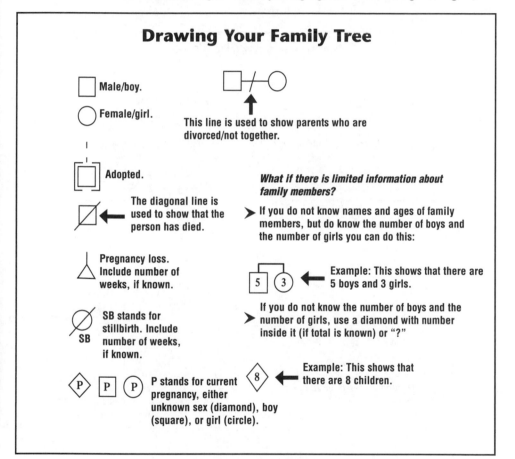

Drawing Your Family Tree

☐ Male/boy.

◯ Female/girl.

This line is used to show parents who are divorced/not together.

☐ Adopted.

⊘ The diagonal line is used to show that the person has died.

△ Pregnancy loss. Include number of weeks, if known.

⊘ SB stands for stillbirth. Include number of weeks, if known.

⬨P ☐P ◯P P stands for current pregnancy, either unknown sex (diamond), boy (square), or girl (circle).

What if there is limited information about family members?

➤ If you do not know names and ages of family members, but do know the number of boys and the number of girls you can do this:

5 ◯3 Example: This shows that there are 5 boys and 3 girls.

➤ If you do not know the number of boys and the number of girls, use a diamond with number inside it (if total is known) or "?"

⬨8 Example: This shows that there are 8 children.

The above illustration shows the basic symbols used in drawing your family tree and family medical history. First, make a list of all of your family members. Then use the sample family tree on page 46 as a guide as you draw your own family tree. Write your name at the top of the paper and the date you drew your family tree. Remember to write your family members' names in place of the words Father, Mother, etc. If possible, draw your brothers and sisters and your parents' brothers and sisters from left to right across the paper, starting with the oldest to the youngest. If dates of birth or ages are not known, just guess as closely as you can.
Illustration reproduced courtesy of the National Society of Genetic Counselors.

For family members with known medical problems, jot down if they smoked, their diet and exercise habits, and if they were overweight. (For example, you could note that your brother John, who had a heart attack at age 40, weighs 300 pounds and smokes two packs a day.)

After you draw your family tree, above your mother's side of the family tree write down where her family members came from (for example, England, Germany, Africa); then do the same for your father's side of the family. This information can be helpful because some genetic health problems occur more often in specific ethnic groups.

Once you've developed your family medical history, share it with your doctors and any genetic caregivers you visit. You may also want to share the information with your relatives.

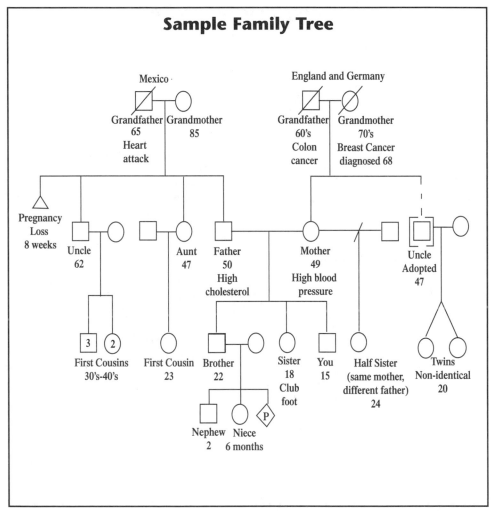

Sample Family Tree

This sample family tree, or pedigree, can serve as a guide to using the symbols shown on page 45 when you draw your own family tree.

Illustration reproduced courtesy of the National Society of Genetic Counselors.

STEP 3: DECIPHER YOUR DNA

As a form of analysis more individualized than family medical history, DNA analysis can give you even more information for your personal genomic blueprint. The number of gene tests is growing rapidly—as of mid-2008, more than 1,300 were available for use in doctor's offices, and many others were available through direct-to-consumer testing companies. All require a DNA sample, and most laboratories can easily extract that from a blood sample. In some circumstances, another tissue sample such as a cheek swab, or a saliva sample, can be used.

These tests can help you find out about a wide variety of conditions, including everything from rare childhood diseases to inherited risks for more common illnesses such as breast cancer. We look in greater detail at specific tests for specific conditions throughout this book. Tests can analyze one specific gene, a variety of genes, or SNPs located throughout your genome. DNA-related tests usually fall into one of the following categories:

- Some diagnose a genetic disease or look for a specific disease-linked gene variant.
- Some determine your risk for disease, but don't offer a firm diagnosis.
- Some focus on a person's identity or ethnic background, for reasons that range from questions of genealogy to answering ancestry questions for adopted children.
- Some focus on research. While these studies are essential to the overall growth of personalized medicine, they may not always provide personal genetic results to individual participants.

Another form of DNA analysis, called genome sequencing, provides a full readout of your entire genome. This type of analysis remains the ultimate goal of DNA testing, and a few individuals, mostly prominent scientists, had had their full genome sequenced. For most of us, however, the cost is prohibitive, especially when scientists still don't know what many parts of the genome do or how they affect health.

Diagnostic Tests

Diagnostic gene tests, the most clear-cut in the personalized medicine toolkit, determine if you carry a disease-linked mutation or set of mutations. While they are most commonly offered after disease symptoms have arisen, diagnostic tests can also be used before you think you might have a genetic illness. If your test uncovers a mutation, you and your doctor may be able to develop a plan of preventive care or medical treatments that limit or stop the mutation's ability to harm your health.

Benefits of diagnostic tests

Diagnostic testing often enables you to discover genetic disease early, or pinpoint the cause of a puzzling ailment. In a family with a high rate of hemochromatosis, or iron overload, for example, a diagnostic test could explain a person's persistent fatigue or painful limbs and allow a doctor to pursue other tests that confirm the presence of the condition. Diagnosis also often brings treatment options. People with confirmed hemochromatosis, for example, can choose to have blood periodically withdrawn from their bodies, lowering their iron levels and preventing iron overload illnesses. (For more information on hemochromatosis, see Chapter 1.)

In other cases, diagnostic tests provide important answers early in life. Some newborns found to have genetic conditions, such as cystic fibrosis, can now receive treatment quickly, whereas they might have developed serious health problems before such tests existed.

Common types of diagnostic tests

Diagnostic testing can now be conducted before a person is even born. In some families where a mutation has already been uncovered, some parents undergoing *in vitro* fertilization (IVF) may choose preimplantation genetic diagnosis (PGD), which assesses an embryo's DNA early in the IVF process. Many would-be mothers now undergo prenatal tests such as amniocentesis, which examines a sample of fetal DNA for genome disorders such as Down syndrome. Newborn babies now undergo blood tests for a wide range of rare but serious genetic disorders shortly after birth. And at any point in life, a person can give a blood sample if they are ill and a disease-linked mutation is suspected as the culprit, or if a genetic condition surfaces in their family. (For more information on pregnancy- and newborn-related diagnostic testing, see Chapter 3.)

Limits of diagnostic tests

In some cases, diagnostic testing may reveal problems for which doctors have few remedies. The discovery of a genetic condition does not always mean the problem can be cured. Expectant parents who learn that their developing baby has the chromosomal abnormality that leads to Down syndrome, for example, have no options for a cure. Instead, they can choose to prepare to welcome their special-needs baby, or end the pregnancy. Some people at risk for carrying the gene for the degenerative and fatal disorder called Huntington's disease choose against diagnostic testing, saying they do not want to learn they have a fatal illness that can't be cured.

Risk Tests

Risk tests are done to look for mutations or SNPs linked to an increased likelihood of genetic disease. These genetic variants do not always mean you'll get sick. Nor are all these tests equally proven. Some risk tests, such as those for certain gene mutations related to breast cancer, have been clearly linked to an increased risk for a disease. Other risk tests, such as some direct-to-consumer tests that analyze your genome for

SNPs related to multiple conditions, are less proven. In many of these cases, DNA may be only one of the factors influencing the occurrence of an illness.

Risk tests can help you understand which health conditions you're more likely to develop, but the test results don't guarantee whether you'll get sick or not. By learning your risks, however, you can follow a preventive health-care plan that reduces your chances of developing an illness tied to a genetic vulnerability or allows you to discover it early, when more treatment options are available to you.

Benefits of risk tests

By revealing genetic risk, this form of testing can guide you toward specific steps you can take to improve your health over the long term.

IT'S YOUR CHOICE

Do You Want a Genetic Test?

Few medical decisions can be more complicated than choosing whether to undergo a genetic test. Genomic experts recommend weighing a broad set of personal questions beforehand, both individually and together with a doctor or genetic counselor. Here are some of them:

- Do you really need this test? What are your chances of having an altered or abnormal gene? If you don't appear to be at risk for having such a gene, the test may only bring unnecessary worry and expense, especially if the answer if not a clear yes or no. For this reason, most doctors do not offer a test unless your family history or other risks show it could really help you.
- What are the possible results of the test? What would a positive result mean for you? Or a negative result?
- What are the advantages of this test? The disadvantages? Will it give you definitive results? How will you feel if it doesn't?
- What do your personal beliefs and values say about testing, or making medical decisions on the basis of test results?
- What will the results mean for your family? Are you comfortable sharing your results with relatives?
- What are your other medical options? Is a test your only choice?
- How long will it take to get your results?
- Who will have access to your test results?
- How much does the test cost? Do you want your health insurance to cover the test and have access to results? Could this test affect your health insurance options in the future? (For more information on insurance, see Chapter 8.)

As you can see from this list of questions, genetic testing touches on much more than one single medical decision. We talk about many of the practical implications of testing, such as privacy and insurance, in Chapter 8.

You might choose to start following preventive health measures such as improving your diet, or undergoing follow-up testing with your doctor to watch for early signs of a condition. In other cases, preventive steps can be more drastic. Some women who take a gene test to detect mutations linked to breast cancer, for example, choose to undergo preventive mastectomy after discovering their risk is much higher than normal.

Those of us who are adopted or don't know at least one of our biological parents may also gain worthwhile insights from this form of testing. Adoptees and others not in contact with their biological family don't know their family health history, and sometimes find that genetic risk testing provides their only way to learn of inherited health risks.

Types of risk tests

Common risk tests include:

- Carrier testing, which examines DNA from would-be parents to see if they have a disease-linked mutation that could be passed on to a child, such as the mutations that cause cystic fibrosis.
- Predictive gene testing, which analyzes your inherited risks for known disease-related mutations, such as those that greatly increase risk for some forms of breast or colon cancer.
- Predictive genomic scans, which analyze many locations on your genome for multiple SNPs related to multiple conditions. These SNPs often carry less risk than the mutations assessed in predictive gene testing, and the results of this form of testing are less definitive.

Limits of risk tests

Increased risk for disease, even when that risk is genetic, does not mean you will become ill. You'll need to examine your results carefully to decide what, if any, action you want to take based on your DNA insights. These types of decisions are best made with the help of a doctor or genetic counselor.

You'll also need to consider the cost of testing. Many risk tests are expensive, and given that they don't always confirm the eventual arrival of disease, doctors and insurance companies may not approve them.

If you sign up with a commercial testing service, be sure you understand how your DNA will be used. At least one such company, for example, shares their customers' DNA with private pharmaceutical and research firms. Established commercial testing companies require that you read and approve an informed consent document prior to purchasing their services. Read through this document carefully to make sure you understand all the ways the company might use your DNA before making a purchase.

Identity Analysis Tests

Identity tests can answer important questions about your background, such as your ancestry or biological relationship to another person. While

If You're Adopted, Or Are Considering Adopting

Adoptees face unique challenges in the era of personalized medicine. They often can't create a family medical history, as they have little or no knowledge of their biological relatives. If you're adopted, or considering adopting a child, here are important steps you can take to uncover as much health information as possible.

Some adoptees are using genetic health arguments to reform state laws that seal adoption records. As of the mid-2000s, seven states—Alabama, Oregon, New Hampshire, Delaware, Tennessee, Kansas, and Alaska—now allow adult adoptees to see their original birth certificate. If you or your adopted child were born in one of those states, you can use the birth certificate information to try to track down biological parents.

For adoptees born in other states, however, the search for birth parents or answers on genetic legacy often remains frustrating. But in some cases, perseverance has paid off. Before Oregon opened its adoption records, for example, a woman named Barbara Casali-Mingus, who had been adopted, knew that one of her adoptive uncles knew the identity of her birth mother. She asked him repeatedly to share the information, finally getting him to relent when she was 31.

Casali-Mingus tracked down her birth mother, only to discover the woman was dying of cervical cancer. While a virus usually causes the disease, genetic factors can increase a woman's risk. At her birth mother's urging, Casali-Mingus went to get screened for cervical cancer, and discovered she too had the disease. After surgery to remove the cancer, Casali-Mingus went on to campaign for more open adoption laws, saying her family discovery probably saved her life.

Some adoptees who can't find their biological family consider undergoing a battery of genetic tests. But most doctors or insurers won't support this option, saying the costly effort may not uncover anything significant. Instead, many doctors recommend that adoptees watch for signs of medical conditions with a genetic link, such as breast cancer at an early age. If you think you're developing a genetic illness, let your doctor know about your adoption history. The unknowns in your family medical history may make your doctors more willing to order relevant genetic tests.

Some adoptive families and adoption agencies have tried to uncover genetic problems at an early age by having young adoptees undergo a battery of genetic screening. But genetic experts recommend against such genetic fishing expeditions, saying they are expensive and can cause psychological harm.

Instead, the American College of Medical Genetics recommends that adoptees be treated as any other children, undergoing routine tests such as newborn screening and further tests only if they appear truly necessary. "The principal objective of genetic testing should be promoting the child's well-being," the recommendation states. "No child brings a guarantee of perfection."

they don't fall within the strict definition of medical testing, identity tests are a growing part of genetic testing and sometimes have health implications. Confirming family relationships or ethnicity, for example, sometimes reveals risks for certain diseases.

Benefits of identity testing

In their most purely informational form, identity tests can answer family questions about ancestry and help people connect with ancestral countries and cultures. For adoptees and others with little knowledge of their family background, identity tests sometimes provide valuable answers about ancestral background health risks. And DNA-based paternity tests can be essential to answering important legal questions.

You may also choose to provide DNA for an identity test that helps identify other members of your family in the event of a tragedy or natural disaster. If you've lost relatives to a natural disaster, for example, your DNA sample could help clarify the identities of the missing as they are discovered. This type of testing, known as forensic testing, lets families recover the remains of loved ones and settle important legal issues such as cause of death and insurance questions.

Common types of identity tests

Identity tests may be conducted either through the study of specific DNA sequences or particular SNPs. A paternity test involving a male child, for example, may compare sections from the Y chromosomes of the boy and the possible father. Ancestry tests often look at SNPs known to have connections to population groups from different parts of the globe.

Limits of identity testing

Not all identity testing is definitive. While paternity testing is often reliable, only certain testing methods are considered admissible as court

---

Did You Know ?

Forensic genetics sounds like detective work—comparing DNA from disaster victims against genes from survivors, looking for a match. But teams of gene experts who stepped in to help find and identify victims after Hurricane Katrina included nurses, doctors, and genetic counselors.

Genetic counselors working at the Louisiana Family Assistance Center, for example, combed through public records to craft family trees for missing persons. Using those trees, the counselors then started dialing all the phone numbers they could find, trying to locate relatives of the missing. In making contact, they'd sometimes find someone who could provide a DNA sample that would help identify the remains of an unidentified victim.

Without the help of these gene experts, it's likely that fewer families would have found the remains of missing loved ones after Hurricane Katrina. These teams also learned lessons that can help the rest of us. Their work bridged "the gap between genetic and forensic medicine to help make our country better prepared to deal with a massive disaster of this nature," said Joan Bailey-Wilson, a scientist who helps lead federal genomic research and coordinated expert help after Katrina.

evidence. If you are considering a paternity test to settle a legal dispute, check with your attorney to make sure you and the test meet all legal paternity testing requirements.

Other types of identity tests have limits as well. Some ancestry or lineage testing may not always provide clear answers, or the company may charge you money to tell you about an ancestral background you already know. Forensic testing may be inconclusive. In some forensic testing done after the World Trade Center attacks in 2001, for example, available DNA fragments were too small or damaged to link victims back to their relatives.

Research Tests

Genomic science can't advance without human DNA to study. As a result, scientists often seek new DNA samples to try to answer large-scale questions about DNA, health, and genetic diseases.

These tests are essential to advances in personalized medicine. Every genomic tool at your disposal started with someone's donated DNA. It is also important to remember that these tests have a goal that goes beyond providing personal genetic information to participants. Some research projects provide DNA results to participants. Others do not.

Benefits of research tests

DNA research is vital to turning knowledge of the human genome into tangible benefits. Advances in genetic care, and better understanding of mutations, polymorphisms, and unique genetic features will not be possible without such research. This is true for the population as a whole, as well as for specific groups. The African-American Biobank at Howard University, for example, was launched in 2003 with the aim of collecting research samples from 25,000 African-Americans so that diseases in that ethnic group could receive their own genomic focus. The Coriell Personalized Medicine Collaborative, mentioned earlier in this chapter, is another example of a large project aiming to gather large amounts of DNA for research. Coriell hopes to enroll 100,000 people in its project and provide individual DNA results to participants.

Common research tests

Some research tests have a narrow focus, such as looking for a mutation or SNP linked to a specific disease. Researchers often find such genetic variants by requesting and taking DNA samples from families known to have a disease, for example, and then analyzing their genes until their mutation is found. Other research efforts are very broad, sifting through millions of SNPs and matching tiny genetic variations with occurrences of disease. One large-scale emerging trend is the type of gene banking mentioned earlier, in which large populations donate samples to be used for a wide variety of experiments over a long period of time.

Limits of research tests

Research is often a slow, uncertain process. In some cases, you may donate samples for research into a particular disease without learning the results for years. Other studies may never provide individual results to participants. If you participate in a research study, you will be asked to sign an informed consent document. Read it carefully to know how your sample will be used and how your privacy will be guarded before making a DNA research or gene bank donation. (For information on genetic privacy issues, see Chapter 8.)

PUTTING DNA KNOWLEDGE TO USE

It's one thing to understand your DNA, and another thing to take action based on what it holds. This next step—putting your genetic insights to good use in individualized ways—is the ultimate goal of personalized medicine. Instead of a one-size-fits-all approach to building health and treating illness, care will become more tailored to the features of your personal genome.

This approach, while still in its early stages, is already redefining some aspects of medicine:

- One promising field of personalized medicine mentioned earlier—drugs that work closely with unique features of individual DNA—is growing rapidly. Pharmacogenomics is rewriting the manual for fighting certain cancers and is beginning to be used in other health fields as well.
- Once they are aware of a person's genetic features, doctors are finding that they can also turn to conventional treatments to counteract the effects of risk-related DNA. Dietary changes, specific types of exercise, and more frequent cancer screenings are just some of the ways that well-established health measures can reduce DNA-related risks.
- Improved genetic understanding is also advancing medicine's ability to work with DNA directly. Researchers, for example, are making notable headway with techniques that block or silence the effects of risk-related genetic variants.

We look more closely at these individual uses of DNA knowledge throughout this book. While DNA insights are only one aspect of your health, genomic experts stress that they can be a powerful ally. Your DNA is not your fate. By understanding it, you can work with it to build better health.

FREQUENTLY ASKED QUESTIONS ABOUT PERSONALIZED MEDICINE

Q. I've downloaded the "My Family Health Portrait" program from the Surgeon General's Web site, and it seems to focus on just a few

Family Tragedy Sparks Changes Toward a Healthier Lifestyle

Fifty-five-year-old Ted was teary on Thanksgiving morning. He was going to celebrate the day with three generations of his family. That was something his father, Steve, never had a chance to do.

Twenty-five years earlier, Ted, then 30 years old, his father Steve, and a few neighbors had gathered for a game of touch football on a beautiful Thanksgiving Day to knock off some of the calories from the holiday dinner. Steve had been running for the goal when he suddenly collapsed. A massive heart attack at age 54 put him in the hospital that afternoon. A week later, Ted was helping his mother plan a funeral.

Steve's heart attack was a replay of the "family curse." Although the family appeared relatively healthy—sure, there was always that extra 15 pounds to lose—it seemed that everyone had heart attacks or strokes before age 60. In fact, the family made a huge deal of birthdays on the 67th year because that was the longest anyone in the family lived. Apparently "longevity genes" didn't run in Ted's family.

The year Steve died, Ted decided to make changes so he was not destined to share the same genetic destiny that had impacted his ancestors. He went to see his doctor, who ran blood tests and diagnosed him with hypercholesterolemia, a condition characterized by high LDL cholesterol. At the time, a molecular genetic test was not available, but the clues were in the family history. Ted will always remember the doctor's comment that if the diagnosis had been made in Steve 30 years earlier, he would still be here.

The same year that Ted discovered he had hypercholesterolemia, he made a serious New Year's resolution to lose weight. He also went on cholesterol-lowering medication. The following Thanksgiving, when the whole family gathered for the first time since Steve's funeral, Ted shared information about hypercholesterolemia with all his aunts, uncles, and cousins, and he encouraged them to see their doctors for this condition. His cholesterol had dropped from a dangerous 514 in February to one that was within normal limits. Ted was on his way to altering the "family curse."

Now, 25 years after Ted lost his father, he was spending Thanksgiving with his entire family, including his oldest daughter who had gotten married two years prior and recently had a baby. By now, the family that gathered for Thanksgiving was larger in number and healthier. By learning who did and did not have hypercholesterolemia, the family was able to change their diets, quit smoking, and take medications as needed. Ted was going to hold his granddaughter today. He planned to spoil her and watch her grow and attend all her ballet recitals–in memory of his father who never had that opportunity.

Bottom Line: As a genetic counselor, I encourage my patients to take advantage of family get-togethers to share information about their relatives' health history. After his father's death, Ted explored the medical reasons for the family health pattern. It would have been easy for Ted to keep his diagnosis to himself, especially after it was well controlled. But as this family learned, knowing both the genetic aspects and the lifestyle of affected family members is important, because lifestyle changes can be life-saving for some conditions.

health conditions. Why? I'm not sure any of these apply to my family.

A. The Surgeon General's family history documents do focus on certain conditions—heart disease, stroke, diabetes, colon cancer, breast cancer, and ovarian cancer. The creators of the program chose these conditions because they are common health problems with a genetic link. They're also conditions you can do something about, through genetic testing or preventive steps to ward off illness. But "My Family Health Portrait" also allows you to enter and track other conditions. You're not limited to these disorders.

Q. *While the federal government is throwing millions of dollars in tax money at scientists to develop personal genome sequences, I have just one thought–"Stop!" What if I don't want my genome sequenced? How will I know how it's going to be stored or used? It feels like scientists are pushing this technology before we even know how to handle the results.*

A. You're not alone in having reservations about the race to sequence individual genomes. Nothing can compel you to have your genome sequenced if you don't want to. In almost all cases, any type of medical testing is entirely voluntary. Standard cholesterol tests, for example, are widely available and highly recommended, but no one can force you take one. The same holds true for genetic tests, and will likely stand for personal genome sequencing, as well.

Q. *Genomic medicine seems to be the only field of health care where I've encountered specialized counselors. Why are genetic counselors necessary? Can't my doctor just talk to me?*

A. As a part of your essential identity, your genes are a far more sensitive and complex topic than almost any other aspect of your health. Genomic medicine touches you, your family, and your future health prospects, often in ways that mix complex gene science with deeply personal decisions. In our hurried system of modern medicine, few doctors have the time or training to talk with patients at length about these issues. Genetic counselors, with training in both the science and emotional effects of genomics, fill that gap.

Q. *I'm thinking about trying a genetic test I saw advertised on a Web site. The company says it is "CLIA certified." Does that mean this company does quality work?*

A. Clinical Laboratory Improvement Act (CLIA) certification applies only to the lab that handles your DNA sample. It says nothing about the quality of the genetic test itself. CLIA certification can't tell you if the test you are considering is accurate or if it analyzes anything truly worthwhile. The best way to ensure that you're getting a quality test is to talk to genetic professionals who've handled many similar tests and cases before.

Q. *What's the point of a risk test? My sister's doctor is suggesting a gene test to assess her chances of inherited breast cancer, but if the test can't give her a definite yes or no answer on whether her cancer is an inherited type, I don't see how it can help. And if she gets the test, do I have to do one too?*

A. You're right—risk tests sometimes only provide limited answers. If your sister gets a definitive "Yes," that information can be extremely useful for her, you, and your other family members. If the answer is "No" or unclear, you may be back to where you started in terms of understanding your risks. The usefulness of risk tests really depends on your own feelings. Some people want any information, even if it's not conclusive. Others don't. Your sister can talk to a genetic counselor before deciding on the test. If she takes the test and finds an inherited risk of cancer, you can make your own decision on whether you want the test as well. The choice is up to you.

Q. *If there are all these genetic tests out there, why don't doctors just offer all of them to everyone? They could probably catch a lot of hidden disease-linked mutations that way.*

A. In theory, widespread testing would uncover unknown genetic risks in some people. But it would also mean running lots of tests on people who don't need them, and cost billions of dollars.

Doctors struggle with this dilemma all the time, even for just one disease. The test for the cancer mutation found in Kevin Lewis, for example, offers valuable health information to people like him and his family. With colon cancer affecting about 150,000 Americans a year, why not offer every colon cancer patient the same test?

Doctors don't, because the numbers don't make it worthwhile. Only about 5 to 10 percent of all colorectal cancers are due to inherited single gene mutations. And at about $3,000, the test is expensive—too expensive to make it worth testing everyone to find such a relatively small number of people at risk, doctors say.

KEEP IN MIND

As you use the tools of personalized medicine to craft a plan for your health that reflects your genes, here are some key points to keep in mind:

- Genomic medicine includes genetic counselors and medical geneticists, specialists who can help you start matching your health care to your genes.
- Personalized medicine can begin with tools as simple as pen and piece of paper for creating a family medical history.
- Some of your DNA can be read and analyzed through genetic tests. Some of these tests offer a clear diagnosis. Others only point out your risk of genetic illness, but can't say definitively whether or not a particular genetic variant will ever make you sick.
- Follow some common-sense guidelines when considering direct-to-consumer genetic tests. Make sure you know how the test works and what its results will tell you. Learn about the company's scientific credentials, and understand how your DNA information will be used. Find out whether the company offers genetic counseling to help you interpret your test results.
- Your DNA is not your fate. If you find that your genome contains risk-related genetic variants, you'll often find a variety of ways to reduce these risks and live a healthier life.

For younger generations, this more personalized approach to better health is now truly a life-long process, starting even before birth. Chapter 3 looks at how genomic advances are changing pregnancy and newborn care.

CHAPTER THREE

YOUR GENES, YOUR PREGNANCY AND YOUR BABY

Diane Guerra and her husband Roy laughed as they dodged a few splashes of water as their kids romped in the backyard wading pool. Their family was happy and boisterous, and the couple was having so much fun raising their children that they were thinking about having one more.

Only one thing was stopping them—Diane's concerns about her age. She was now over 35, the age at which a woman's chances of having a baby with certain birth defects goes up. Diane knew that many other older mothers had undergone genetic testing procedures, such as amniocentesis, to gauge the risk of developmental disorders such as Down syndrome while the baby was still in the womb. But the idea of an invasive test such as an amnio scared her. She personally didn't like the idea of having a big needle inserted into her abdomen to withdraw amniotic fluid, and she was even more concerned about the slight risk of miscarriage that comes with the procedure. But at the same time, she wanted to know as much as possible about the health of their developing baby should she become pregnant again.

Then Diane talked to her doctor, who gave her some good news. She told Diane about a different and more recent procedure that gauges risk for Down syndrome using only a blood sample from the mother and a high-resolution ultrasound image. While not as definitive as an amniocentesis, the results of this screening could still give a strong indication of certain aspects of the baby's health. If the screening raised serious questions, Diane could still opt for an amnio.

Diane, reassured by that option, decided it was time for another baby. She became pregnant a few months later, and the screening test revealed a healthy baby. At the end of the year, she and Roy welcomed another daughter to their family.

This is the fast-changing world of baby making, where scientists are unveiling new innovations that give families more information about the health of their unborn children than ever before. Some families are now selecting the health-related DNA of their next child with the help of fertility clinics that allow families to use embryonic gene analysis. Other labs run tests on hundreds of thousands of fetal gene samples each year, looking for Down syndrome and hundreds of other DNA-related conditions. Expectant parents can find out if they carry risk-related mutations that have been hiding silently in their bodies their entire lives, so that they'll know their risks of passing such a gene on to their baby. And each year, dangerous diseases are spotted in thousands of newborn babies who might otherwise suffer agonizing, mysterious symptoms for months before getting help.

Genomic science has changed the realm of childbearing more dramatically than any other aspect of human health. While genomic care may still be working its way into some other fields of medicine, it has already redefined the world of having babies. Some procedures to check a developing fetus for gene-based illness, such as amniocentesis, have been a routine part of pregnancy care for more than three decades. More recent tests let parents peer into developing embryos just a few cells in size, looking for health problems, desired gender, and sometimes even for a baby with genes that could save the life of an older brother or sister.

This chapter looks at your options for genetic testing while planning for or having a baby, including tests used before, during, and after pregnancy. We also talk about some of the difficult ethical questions surrounding genes and childbearing. While the answers to these questions rest with you, there are important issues you can discuss with your doctor, genetic counselor, partner, or loved ones along the way.

If you are pregnant, or thinking about becoming pregnant, the growth of prenatal and newborn genetic testing makes it likely you'll face at least one or two important decisions related to the health of your baby. Compared to some other aspects of children's health, reproductive genomics receives relatively little oversight from public health officials, so it's a little difficult to say exactly how many pregnancy-related gene procedures are performed each year. But all indications point to a staggering number of genetic tests related to pregnancy and newborn babies, and reproductive genetics now consumes much of the attention of gene specialists and genetic counselors. About four million babies are born in the United States each year, according to federal statistics. Virtually all of those pregnancies and births involve at least some gene-related care—at a minimum, a maternal blood test to check for fetal markers of genetic conditions during pregnancy, and a newborn blood test within days of birth that looks for rare but serious genetic illnesses that require treatment as soon as possible after birth. In 2006, doctors began recommending screening for Down syndrome in every pregnancy.

Expectant mothers who are 35 or older usually undergo the greatest amount of genetic testing—and according to national statistics, more than half a million women a year in that age range now become mothers. This group of women relies more on genetic procedures because of the link between maternal age and gene-related abnormalities in children. Eggs from older mothers are more likely to be aneuploid, meaning they contain an irregular

Did You Know?

The earliest that genes of a human embryo can be analyzed is when that embryo is only eight cells in size.

number of chromosomes. This abnormality sometimes leads to a miscarriage. In other cases, it gives rise to disorders such as Down syndrome. While some individuals with Down syndrome are able to live and grow as independent adults, many still need significant support because of health and developmental concerns.

But the pervasiveness of gene testing during pregnancy doesn't mean that the process is an easy one. Few other life changes pack the emotional complexity of having a baby, and decisions about gene tests and gene-related care add more questions to that journey. Parents face

Making Decisions on DNA Testing During Pregnancy

Genetic testing is now a routine part of prenatal care, but routine hardly means stress-free. This testing involves both you and your developing baby, and touches on deeply emotional issues such as your family history, your hopes for your pregnancy, and your wishes for a healthy baby. Many expectant parents find that genetic testing is one of the most confusing parts of their pregnancy.

Here are issues worth considering as you make your plans for genetic testing during your pregnancy:

- What are your beliefs regarding a baby in different stages of development? Some families, for example, may be more comfortable terminating a pregnancy early if tests reveal a genetic problem in a developing baby, but find themselves reluctant to undergo an abortion later on. Others absolutely oppose abortion in most cases. These considerations can influence the timing of any testing you choose or whether you choose it at all.
- Test results may impact more than just your developing baby. If fetal testing points to a problem, the health of the baby's mother may sometimes also be at risk. Think about how you might choose to weigh the two.
- Think about how you would want to proceed if testing reveals that your baby has a genetic condition. Some families, absolutely opposed to abortion, may still choose to undergo testing so that they can plan for any special medical or developmental needs their baby might have. Others may choose to terminate a pregnancy in that case, but may still need emotional support and help with planning for future pregnancies after such a decision.

As you consider your testing options, seek out a genetic counselor who can help you understand available tests and your options with each of them. Some families also turn to religious advisors, therapists, or close relatives and friends as they make their decisions. For families who elect to continue a pregnancy in which there is a known health concern, special nurses or social workers can be available for counseling through the remainder of the pregnancy, labor and delivery, and for up to 18 months after the birth. Your genetic counselor can identify such a specialist in your community. But remember, no one can force you or your developing baby to undergo or avoid any genetic test. In the end, the decision is up to you.

decisions that affect not only themselves, but also the child they hope to have. For many, the news delivered by gene tests is good, offering happy prospects for a healthy newborn baby. For some others, the news is less hopeful, leaving parents to make painful decisions about their family's fate long before a child is born. Many prenatal gene tests carry conflicting risks that must be weighed against each other, making these medical decisions a complicated balancing act.

Beyond the personal realm, few other areas of genomics are as controversial in our society. As reproductive genomics grows in scope and power, many wonder what comes next—and whether science is heading down an ethical, humane path. Some parents are using PGD solely to select the gender of their next child, a practice many genetic experts find deeply troubling and unethical. Will there also be tests someday to choose a baby's eye color? Height? Intelligence? Will parents be able to build their own designer babies, the way an architect crafts the ideal house? What will happen to embryos, fetuses, and babies deemed undesirable or imperfect?

Public consensus on these questions is scarce. Some privacy advocates say these choices should be left up to families. And advocates in the

Strong Opinions on Reproductive Genomics

When it comes to fertility, Americans have very clear—and very divided—opinions on genomic medicine. Here are a few results from a recent survey involving more than 6,000 people, conducted by Johns Hopkins University's Genetics and Public Policy Center:

- **Appropriate uses.** About two-thirds approved of using prenatal or embryonic testing to diagnose fatal illnesses. But only about half approved of using such technologies for sex selection, and less than one-third approve of their use to look for characteristics such as intelligence or strength.
- **A slippery slope.** More than two-thirds said reproductive genetic technologies will lead to genetic enhancement and designer babies.
- **What reproductive genomics means for society.** Top concerns about social implications included more discrimination against the disabled, less disease research, parents being pressured to use the technology, and loss of genetic diversity.
- **Who should decide.** About two-thirds of participants agreed that such deeply personal decisions should be left to families and individuals. But more than 80 percent also said they were concerned about unregulated reproductive technologies.

These strong public opinions probably reflect those found among your family and friends. As you make your own decisions about your pregnancy, don't be surprised if others want to offer advice. But also remember that these decisions are yours to make, not theirs.

disability community feel that selecting only healthy embryos or fetuses strips society of diversity and compassion—and robs children with developmental differences of their chance at life. A push is growing at the federal level for at least some controls on reproductive gene technologies. As you make your own decisions about your testing and care, you may find yourself buffeted by strong opinions on everything from the ethics of embryonic testing to ending a pregnancy. While these decisions are yours alone, you may sometimes find that sharing them with friends or family brings more disagreement than you would expect—or welcome.

A good place to start reviewing your testing options begins with genetic tests that can be performed long before pregnancy, or even in the first few weeks of your first trimester.

TESTING BEFORE PREGNANCY

Whether you are thinking of having a baby or find yourself newly pregnant, you may want to know if you carry particular genetic risks that could be passed on to a child. We all carry at least a few risk-related genes, and genetic testing can't yet detect all of them. But for certain conditions, you have the option of taking a test to see if you're a carrier—a person with only one copy of a risk-related mutation. That single copy often doesn't harm your health, but if your partner also carries a copy of the same mutation, your children could receive a copy from each of you and develop a genetic illness.

Many obstetricians and prenatal health centers now offer carrier testing that allows you to learn if you carry mutations for particular conditions. Performed on a blood sample, carrier testing can be conducted before or during your pregnancy. If you are pregnant and interested in carrier testing, your doctor will encourage you to take the test early, usually during your first trimester.

Some couples choose carrier testing because they know a particular genetic illness runs in their family. In most cases, however, you are more likely to be offered tests for genetic conditions that arise most often in people who share your ethnic background.

How Carrier Testing Works

Expectant mothers are usually tested first. You give a blood sample at a lab, where your DNA is screened for certain mutations chosen by your doctor. Unless your doctor asks the lab to handle your test quickly, you usually receive your test results within a couple of weeks. If you're an expectant mother who is found to carry a potentially risky recessive mutation, your baby's father will be offered the same test next. If both of you are found to carry the same mutation, your developing baby has a 25 percent chance of inheriting two copies of it. You'll then have the option of undergoing fetal testing that examines your baby's DNA while in utero.

When Carrier Testing Can Help

Here are some of the carrier tests to consider before or during your pregnancy, depending on your ethnicity:

- Sickle cell testing, if you are African-American. Among this group, one in 12 people is a carrier of the sickle cell mutation which causes sickle cell anemia if two copies of the mutation are present. People with sickle cell anemia have misshapen red blood cells that often block small blood vessels, damaging their vital organs and bringing bouts of intense pain.

An Island's Fight Against Thalassemia

Thanks to carrier testing and prenatal genetic testing, the Mediterranean island of Cyprus has turned the tide against a long history of genetic suffering.

Controlled by both Greece and Turkey, Cyprus has a population of more than 700,000 people who share a painful legacy of thalassemia. The form of the condition common on the island, beta thalassemia major, leads to severe anemia, an enlarged spleen, and bone deformities that hamper growth and distort a person's face. Without treatment, many people born with beta thalassemia die by the age of five. Blood transfusions can hold the condition at bay, but they can also result in toxic amounts of iron building up in the body. This iron overload can only be eased by an expensive drug—more than $7,000 per year for an adult—that must be slowly administered several times a week.

On Cyprus, 1 in 7 people carries the beta thalassemia gene, a rate which would normally lead to 1 in 49 marriages occuring between carriers and 1 in 158 babies being born with the disease—about 70 births a year. But only a handful of babies have been born on Cyprus with beta thalassemia major since the mid-1980s. That's because the disease is slowly being eradicated by one of the world's most organized, thorough programs of reproductive gene testing.

Before anyone on Cyprus marries, they must undergo a blood test that reveals whether or not they carry the beta thalassemia major gene. If two carriers marry and become pregnant, they can opt for prenatal testing to see if their developing baby has the disease. If the baby does, the couple can choose to end the pregnancy, with the government covering the cost.

Such an organized campaign to wipe out a disease through widespread gene testing and state-funded abortions might seem controversial. But on Cyprus, support for the program runs high. The demise of thalassemia both reduces suffering and controls health-care costs that would otherwise consume the health budget of the entire island. Families say they have no desire to continue a horrific illness that had inflicted misery on the island for generations. The local Greek Orthodox Church, while rejecting abortion in almost all other circumstances, makes carrier testing part of the process of getting a marriage certificate, and does not oppose the program.

Other countries with high rates of thalassemia, including Pakistan, Singapore, Iran, and the Maldives, have also started preventive testing programs. As these programs grow, it's possible that we'll see the rate of deadly thalassemia continue to fall dramatically around the world.

- Thalassemia testing, if you are of south Asian, southeast Asian, Middle Eastern, or Mediterranean descent. Thalassemia tends to cluster in populations that have historically lived close to the equator on the European, and Asian continents. While carrier rates vary among these groups, as many as one in every seven people is a carrier. The two major forms of the disease, alpha thalassemia and beta thalassemia, arise from mutations on different chromosomes (Chromosome 16 in the case of alpha thalassemia, and Chromosome 11 in the case of beta thalassemia). Both forms give rise to red blood cells that die more easily than normal. Some thalassemia patients need regular blood transfusions to survive. For more information on thalassemia, see Chapter 6.
- Cystic fibrosis (CF) testing, if you are Caucasian, especially if you are of northern or central European descent. Among these groups, one in every 29 people is a carrier of the most common CF mutation, found on Chromosome 7. Two copies of the mutation cause the body to produce abnormally thick, sticky mucus, which clogs the lungs and digestive tract and causes severe breathing and digestive problems. In some people, the effects of cystic fibrosis are relatively mild, while in others, the disease can be fatal at a young age.
- Tay-Sachs testing, if you are a Jew of European descent or a descendant of Canada's and Louisiana's French-speaking populations. Among these groups, about one in every 27 people is a carrier. Two copies of the Tay-Sachs mutation lead to irreversible brain damage. Babies born with Tay-Sachs disease usually die before the age of five. But with the help of carrier testing, health advocates are waging a successful fight against the disease. Over the past 30 years, an organized push to find Tay-Sachs carriers early and limit Tay-Sachs births has reduced the number of cases by about 90 percent, according to federal health statistics.
- Canavan disease testing, if you are a Jew of European descent. Among this group, one in every 40 people is a carrier of the Canavan mutation. Some children born with this degenerative brain disorder die in the first year of life, while others survive into their teens. As with Tay-Sachs disease, an extensive carrier testing program is also driving down the number of babies born with Canavan disease. In the Jewish population, it is also recommended that screening for cystic fibrosis, Gaucher disease, and a developmental disorder called familial dysautonomia be offered.
- As the carrier rate of other genetic diseases is also clarified, some genetic centers are also offering carrier testing for conditions such as Fragile X, which used to be offered only if there was a family history. This condition is different from some others because it is inherited in a sex-linked manner, which means that only the mother would receive screening. A conversation with your doctor will reveal which conditions are currently good carrier testing options for you. For more information on sex-linked disorders, see Chapter 1.

Carrier testing is also available for hundreds of other illness-linked genes. Your doctor, however, is likely to recommend carrier testing for one of these rarer mutations only if a particular illness runs in your family. Here is an example of how that process works for families with a history of a relatively rare disease called spinal muscular atrophy, or SMA. Most people aren't offered carrier testing for SMA, but for SMA families, testing is a routine part of family planning. SMA is a recessive nerve disease linked to mutations found on Chromosome 5. The mutations lead to degeneration of the neurons, or nerve cells, in the spinal cord. The reduction in nerve cells leads to muscle weakness and atrophy, especially in the arms and legs. While some forms of the illness are mild, others can be fatal in children before they reach the age of two.

Gene experts estimate about one in every 40 people is an SMA carrier. That rate is too low for doctors to recommend widespread carrier testing. But families with a history of SMA, or even suspected cases of the disease, usually receive carrier testing when they request it, and share their test results with relatives to see how the SMA-linked mutation appears throughout the family bloodline. If a genetic illness runs in your family, your genetic counselor can help you decide if a similar approach is right for you and your relatives.

Drawbacks to Carrier Testing

When you consider carrier testing, it's important to know that the tests carry some limits. Carrier screening cannot detect every form of a disease-linked mutation. Carrier tests are developed to look for the most common forms of these mutations. That means the tests will detect most of these mutations, but may occasionally miss rare ones. If your carrier test results are negative, that finding greatly reduces your likelihood of being a carrier. But it can't eliminate your risk entirely.

These limits in carrier tests usually become of greater concern if you're seeking a test for a condition less commonly found among people of your ethnicity. The most commonly used carrier tests for conditions such as sickle cell anemia

---

Did You Know **?**

When it comes to cystic fibrosis, your ethnicity says a lot about your risk. Consider the different rates at which people of various ethnic groups carry the most common cystic fibrosis mutation:

- Northern Europeans and Jews of European descent = 1 in 29
- Latinos = 1 in 46
- African-Americans = 1 in 65
- Asian-Americans = 1 in 90

These numbers show why doctors recommend cystic fibrosis carrier testing for people of European descent far more than they do for other groups. But if you are of a different ethnic background, you may still be a good candidate for other versions of the cystic fibrosis carrier test that are more likely to detect different CF mutations occasionally found among others in your ethnic group. Talk to your doctor or genetic counselor about such a test.

or cystic fibrosis, for example, are designed to detect the mutations most commonly seen in ethnic groups that have the highest rates of those diseases. But occasionally, other mutations can cause the same illnesses in people of other ethnic backgrounds. The illness may look the same, but the underlying mutation is different. Commonly used carrier tests often won't be able to detect that rarer mutation. People of every ethnic background develop cystic fibrosis, for example, although not as frequently as Caucasians. Since the most commonly used CF carrier tests look for mutations seen in Caucasians, the same test could miss your CF mutation if you're of a different ethnic background. Talk with your doctor or genetic counselor about how well the available carrier tests suit you, and whether they are likely to detect any mutations you may carry.

Other Considerations for Carrier Testing

If you are already pregnant, and both you and your partner carry the same mutation, you will probably be offered prenatal testing to analyze your developing baby's DNA. Through embryonic or prenatal testing, you have the option of examining your developing baby's genes and risk of genetic disease. Many couples choose this next step, so that they can either plan for the special needs of a child with a genetic illness, or so that they can terminate the pregnancy.

Other couples decide against prenatal testing, saying they would rather take a chance and welcome their new baby "as is" at birth. Your genetic counselor can help you think through each of these options and decide which is right for you.

The Bottom Line on Carrier Testing

Since carrier testing analyzes your genes, not those of a developing baby, it can be conducted at any time before or during your pregnancy. If you're concerned about genetic risks you might pass on to a baby, talk to your doctor about taking a carrier test. You probably won't be tested for every possible mutation, but the test will probably tell you if you carry more common disease-linked mutations.

If you choose to undergo carrier testing and discover that you carry a potentially risky mutation, remember that your future children usually aren't at risk unless your partner carries the same mutation. If both you and your partner are found to be carriers of a particular mutation, and you aren't pregnant yet, you have plenty of time to talk with a genetic counselor about your options for having children.

PRE-IMPLANTATION GENETIC TESTING

If you are eager for a glimpse into the health of a developing embryo, a blend of genomics and fertility science now makes that possible before you are even pregnant.

Pre-implantation genetic diagnosis, or PGD, is an optional part of the process of *in vitro* fertilization. PGD analyzes the genes of an embryo prior to its implantation in a mother's body. The procedure allows expectant parents to select only embryos with desired characteristics in their effort to have a baby. Although PGD cannot guarantee that the baby will be healthy, tests can be performed to evaluate gender or a particular genetic condition, and the implanted embryos will have been chosen because they don't show particular traits. The procedure, first developed is the late 1980s, is still costly and relatively rare. But as PGD techniques have improved, the procedure has become more widespread.

Medical guidelines, such as those established by the American Society for Reproductive Medicine, approve of the use of PGD among would-be mothers with a history of pregnancy-related problems, such as a history of miscarriage or a family history of genetic illness. But in a more controversial shift, PGD is also becoming more popular among families who do not have medical problems but want more choice over their children, especially in selecting a child's gender. In a few other cases, families have undergone PGD to select an embryo for medical reasons, hoping to create a new child who might provide tissues or stem cells to save another family member who is ill. While no one tracks the overall use of PGD, researchers have counted at least 1,000 babies born through the use of PGD, and that number is growing rapidly.

How Pre-Implantation Genetic Diagnosis Works

PGD starts with *in vitro* fertilization, or IVF. A women who undergoes IVF receives hormone injections to stimulate her egg production, and a doctor then removes those eggs from her body. The eggs are mixed with a partner's sperm in the hopes of creating embryos. Once these embryos have grown to several cells in size, a laboratory analyst removes, or biopsies, one or two cells from a developing embryo and conducts an analysis to reveal certain chromosomal or gene abnormalities. This test can also determine the embryo's gender at this time. Expectant parents go over these test results with their doctor, and choose one or several embryos for implantation.

The number of implanted embryos varies from mother to mother, depending on how many eggs were first harvested, how many viable embryos result from *in vitro* fertilization, and how many of those are selected for implantation. Implantation calculations must also balance the parents' comfort with the possibility of multiple births against the chances of a successful pregnancy. A greater number of implanted embryos increases the likelihood of pregnancy, but also raises the chances of twins or triplets if multiple embryos successfully implant. Embryos found to have unhealthy or undesired gene features aren't implanted. Some families opt to keep their unused embryos frozen so that they have the option of implanting them later. Others may choose to donate their unused embryos to other couples unable to conceive on their own, or donate them for research, if possible. Some families decide to have the fertility clinic discard any embryos that aren't implanted.

When PGD Can Help

Some women with a history of miscarriage or problems sustaining a pregnancy are more likely to have a successful IVF pregnancy if they use PGD, researchers say. In addition, this procedure can be of benefit to couples who have an increased chance of having a baby with a genetic

Have a Child, Save a Child

If one of your children suffered from a deadly genetic illness, and the best hope for a cure lay in finding a closely matched tissue or blood donation—preferably from a relative—what would you do? Would you ask all your relatives if they'd be willing to be donors? If none of them provided a good match, would you wait, hoping a donor would emerge from elsewhere?

Or would you follow in the footsteps of some families, who've decided genomic science gives them a choice in addition to waiting? With the help of PGD, would you make your own donor?

In recent years, a small but growing number of parents have decided to have a child to save another. After having one child with a gene-based illness that can only be cured through tissue donation, these parents have opted to have another child designed to be the perfect donor. The process relies on PGD. Embryos created from the parents' sperm and eggs are analyzed to see if they would develop into a child offering a good match to an ailing older sibling. The embryos are also checked to make sure they are free of the same illness that befell the older brother or sister.

Creating these donor babies first made headlines in 2000 with the birth of Adam Nash, a baby boy conceived and chosen to provide a critical transplant for his older sister, Molly. Molly was born with Fanconi anemia, a serious gene-based disease that often kills at a young age. To survive, she needed a successful bone marrow or cord blood transplant—and her odds of survival would increase dramatically if she were to receive a cord blood transplant from a genetically matched sibling. Molly's parents, Jack and Lisa, opted to choose that sibling through PGD. They created and tested 15 embryos before Adam was chosen and born in 2000. Adam provided cord blood for a successful transplant for Molly later that year. Five years later, doctors who performed the transplant at the University of Minnesota said her health remained good.

The Nash case drew plenty of controversy, including accusations that doctors were creating designer babies and forcing infants to be donors without their consent. But families with ailing children argue that their use of PGD in these cases is far from frivolous. The donor babies, they say, are a cherished addition to their families in their own right.

Since Molly's transplant, at least five other infants have been conceived in the United States as donors for a relative. Doctors say the numbers are growing as the use of PGD becomes more widespread.

Genetic Diseases You Can Track with Pre-Implantation Diagnosis

The number of conditions detectable through PGD continues to grow with improvements in gene testing. Here is a partial list of genetic illnesses that have been found through PGD.

If any of these conditions runs in your family, and you are considering having a child, talk to your doctor or genetic counselor.

Aneuploidy disorders (in which a baby inherits an abnormal number of chromosomes)

Trisomy 21 (Down syndrome)
Trisomy 18
Trisomy 13

Single-gene disorders

Adenosine Aminohydrolase (ADA) Deficiency
Adrenoleukodystrophy (X-Linked ALD)
Alpha 1 Antitrypsin Deficiency
Alpha-L-Iduronidase (IDUA)
Alport Syndrome (X-Linked)
Ataxia-Telangiectasia
Basal Cell Nevus Syndrome (Gorlin Syndrome)
Blepharophimosis, Ptosis, and Epicanthus Inversus (BPES)
Blood Group—Kell Cellano System
Brain Tumor, Posterior Fossa of Infancy, Familial
Ceriod Lipofuscinosis, Neuronal 2. LAE Infantile. CLN2 (Batten Disease)
Charcot-Marie-Tooth Disease Type 1A (CMT1A)
Charcot-Marie-Tooth Disease Type 1B (CMT1B)
Charcot-Marie-Tooth Disease, Axonal, Type 2E
Charcot-Marie-Tooth Disease, Type X-Linked, 1 (CMTX1)
Choroideremia (CHM)
Citrullinemia, Classic
Congenital Adrenal Hyperplasia (CAH)
Crouzon Syndrome (Craniofacial Dysostosis)
Currarino Triad
Cystic Fibrosis (CF)
Cystinosin (CTNS)
Darier-White Disease (DAR)
Diamond-Blackfan Anemia (RPS19)
Dystonia Torsion (DYT1)
Early-Onset Familal Alzheimer Disease
Ectodermal Dysplasia 1, Anhidrotic (ED1)
Emery-Dreifuss Muscular Dystrophy, Autosomal Dominant (EDMD3)
Emery-Dreifuss Muscular Dystrophy, Autosomal Recessive (EDMD3)
Epidermolysis Bullosa Dystrophica, Pasini
Epiphyseal Dysplasia, Multiple, 1 (EDM1)
Exostoses, Multiple, Type 1
Fabry Disease
Familial Adenomatosis Polyposis
Familial Dysautonomia (Riley-Day Syndrome, DYS)
Fanconi Anemia A
Fanconi Anemia C
Fragile X A Syndromes (FMR1)
Galactosemia
Gaucher Disease, Type 1

Glycogen Storage Disease, Type VI
Hemophilia A
Hemophilia B
Diamond-Blackfan Anemia (DBA)
Holoprosencephaly
Hunter Syndrome (Mucopolysaccharidosis II)
Huntington Chorea
Hurler Syndrome (Mucopolysaccharidosis I)
Hydrocephalus, X-Linked (L1CAM)
Hoyeraal-Hreidarsson Syndrome (HHS)
Hypophosphatasia (Infantile)
Immunodeficiency with Hyper-IgM, Type 1
Incontinentia Pigmenti (IP)
Krabbe Disease
Li-Fraumeni Syndrome
Long-Chain Hydroxyacyl-CoA Dehydrogenase (HADHA)
Marfan Syndrome
Metachromatic Luekodystropy
5,10-@Methylenetetrahydrofolate Reductase (MTHFR)
Mucopolysaccharidosis, Type 2
Muscular Dystrophy, Duchenne Type (DMD)
Muscular Dystrophy, Becker Type (BMD)
Myotonic Dystrophy (DM1)
Myotubular Myopathy 1
Neurofibromatosis, Type 1
Neurofibromatosis, Type
Norrie Disease
Oculocutaneous Albinism
Oculocutaneous Albinism, Type 2
Omenn Syndrome
Optic Atrophy
Ornithine Carbamoyltransferase (OTC) Deficiency
Osteogenesis Imperfecta (Col1A1,Col1A2)
Osteopetrosis, Malignant, Autosomal Recessive
Pelizaes-Merzbacher Disease
Phenylketonuria (PKU)
Polycystic Kidney Disease Autosomal Dominant, Type 1
Polycystic Kidney Disease Autosomal Dominant, Type 2
Polycystic Kidney Disease Autosomal Recessive
Retinitis Pigmentosa
Retinoblastoma (RB1)
Rett Syndrome
Sandhoff Disease
Sickle Cell Anemia
Spinal Muscular Atrophy (SMA)
Spinocerebellar Ataxia, Type 1
Spinocerebellar Ataxia, Type 2
Spinocerebellar Ataxia, Type 3 (also known as Machado-Joseph Disease)
Spinocerebellar Ataxia, Type 6
Spinocerebellar Ataxia, Type 7
Symphalangism Proximal (SYM1)
Tay-Sachs Disease (TSD)
Thalassemia Alpha
Thalassemia Beta
Treacher Collins Syndrome
Tuberous Sclerosis, Type 1
Tuberous Sclerosis, Type 2
Von Hippel-Lindau Syndrome (VHL)
Zellweger Syndrome

condition but don't want to face an abortion decision later in the pregnancy. But the procedure still doesn't guarantee the birth of a healthy baby—or even a baby at all. Two PGD studies, for example, found that about 30 to 35 percent of PGD implantations resulted in pregnancy.

In a few cases, families have turned to PGD to create a child who could save another. In these families, one child had been diagnosed with a serious illness, such as life-threatening anemia, that is best cured with a carefully matched tissue donation. These families have used PGD to select a baby who can provide the right match to save their big brother or sister.

The Drawbacks of PGD

There is no agency overseeing the accuracy or safety of PGD, leaving few ways to reliably track its success rates or results. Doctors who offer it say PGD usually works correctly in revealing gender and detecting risk-related DNA. But some research groups, such as the Genetics and Public Policy Center at Johns Hopkins University, have reported that in a small number of cases, PGD failed to reveal the genetic abnormality the screening was intended to detect. Similar questions surround the safety of harvesting a cell or two from a developing embryo. Many IVF practitioners say such a biopsy, usually done when an embryo is between four and 10 cells in size, is safe and does not harm the developing embryo. But so far, no one has consistently tracked the health of children born after a PGD procedure. If you are considering PGD, talk to fertility clinics about their safety procedures, experience, and success rates. Some clinics are far more experienced with PGD than others.

Other Considerations for PGD

Few practices in genomic medicine are more controversial than PGD for gender selection. Many professional societies and doctors now support PGD for families with a history of genetic illness or women with a history of miscarriage or other pregnancy problems. But the growth of PGD as a tool for simply choosing between a baby boy or girl has left some ethicists and lawmakers questioning whether the procedure should be more tightly controlled. If you are interested in PGD for gender-selection purposes, here are some important points to keep in mind:

- Using PGD purely as a tool for sex selection is allowed in the United States but prohibited in some other countries, including Canada and Great Britain.
- In the United States, private clinics are more likely to offer PGD analysis for the purpose of gender selection, saying such choices should be left up to families. But reputable academic medical centers are less likely to offer PGD as a way to choose a baby boy or girl, saying PGD should only be used to screen embryos for genetic

illness. Some only offer sex selection to families with a known history of gender-linked gene disorders, such as hemophilia and Duchenne muscular dystrophy. Since the mutations that cause many of these gender-linked gene disorders can be analyzed in detail, the records of the previously affected child can be stored, and will help the clinic and the family make PGD decisions using the most accurate information available.

- PGD is expensive. One round of PGD and IVF can cost well over $15,000, with no guarantee of the procedure producing a healthy pregnancy. Insurance coverage is rare, though insurance companies may be more likely to cover some of the cost in cases of a confirmed family history of genetic illness.
- PGD and IVF can also be uncomfortable for the mother. IVF is an elaborate process that usually includes hormone injections, egg harvesting, and embryo implantation. Many women experience uncomfortable side effects during the process, including pain, moodiness, and bloating due to the hormone shots used to stimulate release of eggs.

The Bottom Line on PGD

If you are interested in PGD, start by talking with your family doctor or obstetrician. If you're interested solely for the purpose of picking your baby's gender, however, remember that many people think the practice is unethical. Many doctors, medical centers and fertility clinics won't be willing to help you. Keep the costs and important ethical questions that come with PGD in mind as you decide whether it's the right choice for your family.

TESTING YOUR DEVELOPING BABY

Gene screening during pregnancy is now a routine part of most prenatal care. Prenatal testing allows you to learn whether your developing baby has certain genetic abnormalities or illnesses. Some of these tests only require an image of your baby and a sample of your blood,

Did You Know?

Scientists around the world are working to develop a new type of prenatal test that requires nothing more invasive than drawing a blood sample from an expectant mother.

When you are pregnant, cells and free-floating bits of DNA from your developing baby enter your blood stream and circulate through your body. Scientists in the United States, Hong Kong, and Europe are now working on ways to remove and screen enough of these cells to reveal the same genomic information now gleaned from tests such as amniocentesis.

So far, this method has proven far less accurate than current prenatal tests. It can only detect up to 75 percent of Down syndrome cases, compared to a detection rate of almost 100 percent for amniocentesis. But the research continues as scientists work to improve the test, and some scientists say this form of testing might be available some time after 2010.

which is analyzed to see if it contains substances linked to developing babies with genetic problems. Others require a sample of your developing baby's DNA, usually obtained by taking a bit of the tissue or fluid that surrounds the baby in your uterus.

Prenatal tests fall into two categories: predictive screening and diagnostic testing. Almost all prenatal tests are performed in the first or second trimester.

How Predictive Screening Works

Predictive screening tests can indicate an increased risk for conditions such as Down syndrome. Some predictive screening is conducted by using ultrasound, a non-invasive imaging technology that creates images of your developing baby. Another common form of predictive screening measures substances in the mother's blood—usually a marker called alpha-fetoprotein (AFP) and hormones such as estriol or human chorionic gonadotropin—that may also indicate an increased risk for conditions such as Down syndrome if they're present at levels different from the norm. This blood test is commonly referred to as maternal serum screen, and additional markers are being studied and included as they show improved evaluation of the developing fetus.

One more recent predictive test, the nuchal translucency or NT ultrasound, combines the ultrasound and the blood test into one that is more accurate than using the two separately. The ultrasound measures the nuchal fold, an area at the back of your developing baby's neck. In the early weeks of your pregnancy, the thickness of this fold is often related to the presence of Down syndrome. Together with a maternal serum screen, the NT ultrasound has the ability to detect more than 90 percent of Down syndrome cases. Once usually used mostly in women older than 35, recent changes to medical recommendations now make the NT ultrasound available to expectant mothers of any age. This is the type of screening chosen by the Guerra family, whose story we introduced at the start of this chapter.

The Drawbacks of Predictive Screening

Predictive screening is designed to identify women who may have higher-risk pregnancies, not to provide a firm diagnosis. Therefore, screening is typically not accurate enough to conclusively pinpoint gene-based illness. Blood tests alone, especially the maternal serum screen, have a high rate of false positive results, meaning they indicate problems where none actually exist. For this reason, your doctor will recommend further testing if your maternal screen points to a problem.

The NT ultrasound, together with a blood test, has proven more accurate than regular ultrasound or blood tests alone. But it usually must be performed early in the pregnancy. And not all health-care providers offer the NT ultrasound yet, as a specially trained technician must perform the procedure. If you are interested in an NT ultrasound, talk to your obstetrician about getting an early referral to a hospital or medical center that offers NT ultrasound, so that you can get the test before your pregnancy is too advanced for the test to be worthwhile.

Other Considerations for Predictive Screening

Most insurance plans previously covered the costs of NT ultrasound for mothers over 35. But recent changes to medical recommendations should make more insurance carriers willing to cover the cost for any woman whose plan includes maternity benefits, regardless of age. As part of your preparation for the test, find out your insurance company's policy on NT ultrasound ahead of time.

The Bottom Line on Predictive Screening

Predictive screening often offers a good first glimpse into your developing baby's risk of genetic disease. But if you want definitive answers, you may not find some of these tests to be conclusive enough. The big exception to this is the NT ultrasound, which is an increasingly popular option for women who don't like the risks that come with more invasive types of testing. Talk with your doctor or genetic counselor early about the best testing options to fit your family history, stage of pregnancy, and level of comfort with genetic tests.

DIAGNOSTIC TESTING

Diagnostic testing is more accurate than predictive testing, but also more invasive. The most accurate diagnostic test is amniocentesis, often referred to as an amnio. In amniocentesis, a doctor removes a sample of fetal cells by inserting a long needle through the mother's abdomen and into the uterus, taking a sample of amniotic fluid. Fetal cells float in the fluid, and after removal and further growth in a lab, the chromosomes or DNA from the fetus can be analyzed using the same methods common for other types of gene analysis. Parents must often wait up to two weeks for test results, although the faster, less accurate analysis known as fluorescence *in situ* hybridization (or FISH) can often offer preliminary results within a few days. Amniotic fluid can be analyzed to reveal almost all chromosomal disorders, including Down syndrome, gene-based illnesses such as cystic fibrosis, and neural tube defects such as spinal bifida. Doctors typically recommend having the test between the 15th and 20th weeks of pregnancy.

Another common diagnostic test, chorionic villi sampling (CVS), uses a syringe and catheter to remove a small sample of tissue that connects the amniotic sac to the wall of the uterus. The makeup of this tissue typically matches that of the fetus, providing cells for DNA analysis. CVS can reveal many of the same disorders as amniocentesis, including Down syndrome, although it cannot detect spina bifida. Results may take up to 10 days, although preliminary results may sometimes be available more quickly. A CVS is typically done between 10 and 12 weeks into a pregnancy. For some women, this earlier testing time makes CVS an attractive choice.

Doctors may also occasionally recommend other invasive diagnostic tests, such as umbilical blood sampling. In this test, a small amount of fetal blood is drawn from the spot where the baby's umbilical cord attaches to the placenta, providing a tissue sample for DNA testing. This procedure is usually offered only if reliable information cannot be obtained through more common tests such as amniocentesis.

The Drawbacks of Diagnostic Testing

While diagnostic tests are usually accurate, amniocentesis has proven slightly more accurate than CVS. The CVS test occasionally returns unclear results, preventing your doctor from using the test to determine whether your developing baby has significant genetic abnormalities. Women who receive a questionable CVS result are usually referred for a follow-up amniocentesis.

Both procedures involve inserting a needle or probe into the uterus, which poses a small risk to your pregnancy. According to the federal health statistics, the risk of miscarriage from CVS is between 1 in 100 and 1 in 200. The risk of miscarriage from amniocentesis is lower—about 1 in 1,600. In both cases, risks are closely tied to the experience and skills of the medical practitioners performing the tests. Ask the doctors performing your CVS or amniocentesis how many such procedures they've done in the past, and whether any miscarriages have resulted among their patients.

Other Considerations for Diagnostic Testing

Because of the small risk of miscarriage associated with diagnostic testing, these tests are usually only offered when you have a greater need for them. Mothers over 35 routinely are offered diagnostic testing, although as noninvasive tests improve, this may change. If you are younger than 35, you're only likely to be offered diagnostic tests if the results of your predictive screening tests, such as your maternal serum screen or NT ultrasound, indicate that your baby may be at greater risk for a genetic abnormality.

In some cases, expectant parents decide against any diagnostic testing. Some aren't comfortable with the risks. Some decide they would prefer to find out how healthy their baby is at birth. Others look at all the odds in their favor, and decide testing isn't worth it. About 95 percent of amniocentesis tests, for example, reveal developing babies with no detectable problems. And the vast majority of babies are born healthy, regardless of whether or not they were tested.

If your testing does detect a problem, it's important to remember that there may be little you can do to treat your developing baby. Except in a few cases, genetic illness cannot be corrected in utero or cured after birth.

If your testing detects an abnormality or illness, you may choose to have an abortion. Or you may decide to have your baby, and use your test results to start planning for any special care your baby may need.

Expectant Couple Struggles with Possibility of Down Syndrome Baby

Kelly was at home relaxing because this pregnancy was tougher than her first one 8 years ago. Her two previous miscarriages also increased her nervousness, even though she *was* 17 weeks along, 6 weeks further than the latest miscarriage. Then the phone rang with some devastating news.

It was the office nurse, telling her that the blood test from her last visit was abnormal and that meant that the baby might have Down syndrome (DS). Kelly was told to see a genetic counselor and given a phone number to make an appointment. It couldn't be true. Kelly couldn't stop crying, but finally brought herself under control and called her husband. She could barely get the words out, so Dan called the doctor's office and then the counselor to make an appointment the next day.

After a sleepless night, Kelly and Dan, who had spent the night on the Internet reading about DS, met with Susan, the genetic counselor. She clearly had lots of experience with anxious parents. They spent the first 10 minutes discussing how important this pregnancy was, their daughter who was so looking forward to a new sibling, and their fears because of the miscarriages. Susan then asked about the pregnancy and family history.

The pregnancy history did not increase any risks for the baby, although Susan asked lots of questions about the miscarriages. The most important information turned out to be the maternal serum screen, which indicated that there was a higher chance that the baby might have DS. She also told them about the ultrasound and amniocentesis that could provide more definitive information. Whoa. The ultrasound sounded okay, but the amnio involved a needle. And even though the doctor had lots of experience, Kelly didn't want *any* risk of a miscarriage. Dan wasn't so sure—a baby with DS would take a lot of resources and energy he wasn't sure they had. Susan spent some time talking about children with DS and offered to introduce the couple to some families with DS children.

Susan then spent time helping both of them balance reasons for and against an amnio. In the end, many of Dan's concerns were eased, and Susan supported their decision to have an ultrasound, but no amnio. Susan knew that they would worry, so she offered a strategy to put the risk in perspective. After the ultrasound, it was determined that the risk of having a baby with DS was 1 in 100. So Susan asked them to spend one of every 100 hours preparing for a baby with DS. The other 99 hours should be spent preparing for a normal baby—who would grow up to be a teenager wanting driving lessons!

Bottom Line: As a genetic counselor, I encourage my patients to make the decision that works for them. They will receive lots of advice from family, friends, neighbors and other health care providers, but they are the ones who have to live with the decision, so my role is to ensure that it is one that works with their life experience and value system. All Kelly and Dan's prep work ultimately left them in good shape to greet their healthy baby, who did not have Down syndrome.

The Bottom Line on Diagnostic Testing

Diagnostic testing can offer you lots of answers about your baby's health. But it also carries more risks than other forms of prenatal testing.

Part of your decision on diagnostic testing will likely involve the age of the mother and timing of the test. Some mothers who choose diagnostic testing opt for a CVS because it can be done earlier, even though the procedure carries a little more risk. Others wait for an amniocentesis to lower their risk of complications or miscarriage. Your options will probably depend, in part, on when you receive the results of your earlier predictive screening tests.

Talking with a genetic counselor is especially helpful when you are deciding on diagnostic testing. Counselors have detailed information on the risks of various procedures and can help you compare one procedure against another. Is an NT ultrasound that detects up to 90 percent of Down syndrome cases and carries no risk to your baby, for example, as good as an amniocentesis that detects almost 100 percent of cases but carries a small risk of miscarriage? When you're trying to balance one set of risks against another, a counselor's experience can be invaluable. A genetic counselor can help you weigh testing risks in your own situation and help you make the decision that is right for you.

TESTING YOUR NEWBORN BABY

Once your baby is born, your busy first few days as a new parent will probably include your child's first encounter with genomic medicine.

Almost all babies born in the United States now undergo a round of gene-related newborn screening tests shortly after birth. Performed using a few drops of blood drawn from your baby's heel, the testing is designed to catch genetic disorders that are otherwise difficult to diagnose and can cause serious health and developmental problems. According to the federal Centers for Disease Control and Prevention, about 3,000 babies in the United States each year are found to have severe disorders detected through newborn screening.

Newborn screening usually looks for metabolic disorders, in which a DNA doesn't allow the body to process nutrients correctly. While these conditions are rare, arising in only one out of every several thousand births, their effects can be devastating. Such metabolic problems, such as phenylketonuria, often lead to serious illness or developmental

> ## *Did You Know* ?
>
> The March of Dimes, a major national non-profit advocacy group working to prevent birth defects, organizes public campaigns to improve newborn screening in states with weaker screening programs. If you'd like to find out more about newborn screening in your state, or get involved in urging your lawmakers to create a more thorough screening program, visit the group's Web site at www.marchofdimes.org and click on the Pregnancy and Newborn section.

damage. Others, such as a condition called galactosemia, are fatal if left untreated. A look at galactosemia, one of the conditions commonly assessed during newborn screening, shows how these disorders usually occur and unfold. Galactosemia is caused by variations in the *GALT* gene, which carries the code for an enzyme critical to processing galactose, one of the main sugars in milk. Without the correct version of this enzyme, babies cannot properly metabolize galactose. Unhealthy levels of galactose build up in their bodies and cause severe damage to the liver, nervous system, and other organs. Since infants are normally fed milk rich in galactose, the disorder must be caught quickly—often within 10 days—to prevent the most serious and potentially fatal long-term health problems associated with the condition. Symptoms of galactosemia include jaundice, an enlarged or damaged liver, and vomiting, but the best way to catch the disease is through newborn screening. Children with the condition must be fed lactose-free formula and avoid dairy products throughout their life. Even then, they remain at risk for developmental delays and speech problems, depending on when their condition was diagnosed.

Phenylketonuria, or PKU, is also a frequent part of newborn screening. For more information on PKU, see Chapter 4.

How Newborn Screening Works

Shortly after your baby's birth, a nurse will prick your baby's heel and collect a few drops of blood using a special absorbent paper card. The contents of these drops are then analyzed to see if they show levels of metabolic compounds linked to certain metabolic disorders.

State public health departments usually set the rules for newborn screening programs, with each state choosing which conditions will be covered by the testing. As a result, the number of conditions included in newborn screening varies widely from state to state. The number of conditions covered by each state, however, has increased in recent years, and many states now test for more than 30 conditions. As of mid-2008, all states offered newborn screening for seven conditions, including PKU, a range of sickle-cell diseases, congenital hypothyroidism, and galactosemia. Ask your obstetrician or pediatrician about the conditions covered by newborn screening in your state.

When Newborn Screening Can Help

If your baby's newborn screening test indicates that your baby has a metabolic disorder, the information can literally be a lifesaver. Since many of the conditions detected through newborn screening can be managed by controlling a child's diet, restricting or eliminating a problem nutrient can limit or prevent the damaging effects of a metabolic disorder. But such steps must often be taken in the first days or weeks of life to prevent problems. That's why the early information provided by newborn screening is so important.

If your baby's screening results point to a problem, your doctor may refer you to a metabolic specialist immediately and put your baby on a restricted diet. Your doctor may also recommend further genetic testing to confirm the diagnosis and refer you to a genetic counselor.

The Limits of Newborn Screening

In some cases, however, dietary controls may offer only limited help. The range of treatment options varies greatly between different metabolic disorders. Your doctors will help you develop a diet for your baby that is most likely to limit or prevent damage from a metabolic disorder.

Because newborn screening is just that—an initial scan, not a complete diagnosis—occasionally, it returns a false positive result. In these

A Family's Fight for Newborn Screening

After one of her babies died in the middle of the night, Deborah Houk vowed she wouldn't lose her next.

Late in the summer of 1990, the young mother and nurse from Tempe, Arizona, was pregnant with her third child, her family's first boy. But excitement over the new baby bumped up against a heart full of grief. Houk's second child, a bubbly, energetic 18-month-old girl named Lauren, had died mysteriously in her sleep about eight months before.

The Houks and their doctors were baffled by Lauren's death. The toddler and her older sister Meghan were both suffering from a bout of the stomach flu when Lauren died. Both girls had upset stomachs, and had been sipping clear fluids instead of eating much. But stomach flu is a routine part of childhood, and Lauren had seemed fine when her parents last checked her at midnight. Early the next morning, her father went to wake her.

"The next thing I knew, my husband was running screaming down the hallway," Houk remembers. "I knew something was really wrong. From the sound of his voice, I knew she was dead."

Doctors and the coroner suggested that Lauren had succumbed to some type of sudden infant death syndrome. But her mother couldn't believe that. Lauren seemed too old for such a problem, which often strikes infants in the first few months of life. Houk instinctively thought something genetic might be at play. She wanted to protect her next baby, and underwent an amniocentesis. But that screening found nothing unusual.

Then she got a phone call from the coroner.

A colleague in California had sent him a medical article on a genetic condition called MCADD, or Medium Chain Acyl-CoA Dehydrogenase Deficiency. The rare hereditary disease leaves a person without an enzyme that converts fat into energy. People with MCADD seem perfectly healthy, until a problem like the stomach flu leaves them unable to eat. Without steady food, their bodies fail quickly. Most of MCADD's victims are small children, who show no signs of their cases, your baby is actually healthy, but you receive test results that indicate the possible presence of a metabolic disorder. False positives are uncommon in newborn screening, however, and the follow-up testing that comes after an initial diagnosis will reveal the error in the initial test.

Other Considerations for Newborn Screening

State health departments encourage newborn screening for all infants, but many also allow families to request an exemption for religious reasons. In most states, the test is done routinely, and often parents are not even aware that it happened unless they receive a call that the screening shows an abnormality.

While most insurance providers now cover newborn screening, a few may not. Check with your insurance carrier prior to your baby's birth.

condition until a minor ailment leaves their stomachs empty for an extended period of time.

Houk talked to her obstetrician. "I think Lauren died from MCADD," she told him, "and I have another baby on the way." He replied that she was worrying needlessly. She considered his advice—and then decided to act on her own. She tracked down MCADD researchers, and had the coroner send a tissue sample from Lauren for testing.

The sample showed Lauren had MCADD. The recessive illness, caused by a gene mutation on Chromosome 1, had a 25-percent chance of striking each of the Houks' children. Meghan tested negative for the disease, although she is a carrier like her parents. But what about the baby on the way?

Broad newborn screening programs weren't in place at that time. But the Houks ordered a special kit so that their son, Austin, could be tested right after his birth in late 1990. Within a week of Austin's arrival, the Houks learned he also had MCADD. The knowledge let the family take important medical steps to help Austin, such as giving him fluids intravenously when he came down with the flu, ear infections, or other childhood ailments.

Now a thriving, healthy teenager, Austin is a star student and athlete. His mother has turned her family's struggle into a public campaign, pushing for the expansion of Arizona's newborn screening program. Recently, her efforts paid off. As of 2006, the state, which once lagged in newborn screening, expanded its testing to cover almost 30 conditions.

Houk also advises other families, urging them to be persistent and thorough when it comes to their children's genes and health. "Find out about the extent of screening in your state," she says. "Order supplemental screening if your state's testing falls short. If your pediatrician questions the value of screening, find one more supportive of your knowledge and decisions.

"If we had not pursued things on our own, we would have wound up in a much worse place," Houk says. "Don't take 'No' for an answer. Ever."

If your state offers only limited newborn screening, many pediatricians will conduct a more thorough test if you ask. Before your child's birth, check with your pediatrician about the range of tests offered in your state and what broader testing options your doctor recommends. Many pediatricians offer supplemental testing themselves, arranging for extra testing in the hospital after a baby's birth. If your doctor won't arrange for supplemental testing, you can order a broader newborn screening kit yourself and have your doctor or hospital conduct the test for you. These kits can be ordered from a variety of sources, including Baylor Health Care System (www.baylorhealth.com) and Pediatrix (www.pediatrix.com). These kits cost anywhere from $25 to almost $100. Genetic experts recommend that these supplemental kits be ordered well before your baby's birth, so that testing can be conducted in the hospital shortly after your baby arrives.

The Bottom Line on Newborn Screening

Unless you object to newborn screening on religious grounds, most gene experts and pediatricians strongly recommend this test for your baby. It's easy and inexpensive. And while the problems it detects are rare, the test can give you life-saving information early if your baby does have metabolic disorder.

FREQUENTLY ASKED QUESTIONS ON GENES AND PREGNANCY

Q. I'm interested in using PGD to make sure our next baby is a boy. But when I checked into the price, it would probably cost more than $15,000! And our insurance company says they won't help pay. Why is PGD so expensive, and why won't our insurance help us?

A. PGD often costs that much or more, in part because the procedure is complicated. It involves more than just gene analysis, requiring all the hormones and steps that go with *in vitro* fertilization. And fertility clinics that offer PGD as a tool for gender selection are usually for-profit establishments. They know people who really want to select the sex of their baby will pay for the privilege, and they set their prices accordingly.

Gender selection is a parental preference, not a medical concern. Therefore, since insurance companies deal with medical concerns, most won't cover it.

Q. I'm Asian-American, and my husband is white. Does that difference affect which carrier tests we should take before getting pregnant?

A. Your testing situation may be a little more complex, but your different backgrounds can also benefit your baby genetically. As a woman interested in being a mother, you'll usually take a carrier test before your husband does. You'll be tested for any conditions known to be prevalent in your ethnic group. In your case, that would be the thalassemias. If your test shows any results of concern, your husband will be tested, as well. He'll probably be tested for the same conditions, as you were, along with any conditions more prevalent in his ethnic group, such as cystic fibrosis. Then if he were a CF carrier, you would be tested for that, as well. Your baby would only be at increased risk for genetic illness if both of you are shown to carry the same risk-related mutation. Here, your different backgrounds work to your advantage, making it less likely the two of you share an ethnically linked mutation.

Q. *One of my friends got an ultrasound picture of her baby at a local shopping mall. Everything looked great—he was so cute! Now her doctor wants her to have another ultrasound. Can too many ultrasounds cause any damage to the developing baby?*

A. Having another ultrasound won't cause any harm to the baby, and is actually a good idea for both the baby and his mother's health. Ultrasounds done at the mall are great fun, but they usually come with a waiver you have to sign saying that no medical information would be provided as part of the scan. Though the picture is cute, it doesn't offer any useful information about the baby's health. The ultrasound that your friend's doctor wants to do will be medically helpful, conducted by experts trained at spotting problems and reviewed by a physician. While some ultrasound centers in hospitals also provide keepsake photos for parents, the two procedures' purposes are quite different.

Q. *Before I got pregnant, I thought prenatal testing sounded like a great idea. But now, I'm not so sure. I'm worried about the risk of miscarriage that comes with an amniocentesis. Do I have to undergo one?*

A. No, you don't. No one can force you to undergo an invasive prenatal test. There are certain situations in which your doctor or genetic counselor may recommend testing more strongly, such as if your blood test reveals a potential concern or if a genetic illness runs in your family. Predictive tests, such as an NT ultrasound, also help you get a better sense of risks facing your developing baby and help you decide whether you think invasive testing is necessary.

Q. *I'm 27 and expecting my first baby. I'd always thought amniocentesis was for older moms, but after I took an AFP test, my doctor says my results show that an amnio is a good idea. What's going on? I thought younger mothers didn't have to worry about this.*

A. You're right about the typical age for amniocentesis—the procedure isn't routine for mothers younger than 35. But your age only reduces your baby's risk of gene-related problems. Being younger can't eliminate that entirely. But also remember that the AFP test sometimes returns false positive results. Talk with a genetic counselor about your AFP results, what risks they indicate, and the AFP's false positive rate in cases such as yours. That information can help you decide whether an amniocentesis is something you want to pursue next.

Q. *My state's newborn screening only tests for a few conditions. I'd like to order a supplemental screening kit, but the pediatrician I'm considering as my baby's doctor says it's not necessary. What's the best thing to do?*

A. In discouraging you from supplemental screening, the pediatrician you are interviewing is probably reacting to the fact that many of the metabolic disorders detected by newborn screening are rare. While that's true, most gene experts would also say that avoiding supplemental testing for that reason is misguided. Supplemental screening is quick, easy, and inexpensive. Even if these metabolic disorders are unusual, why not find out for sure? If this pediatrician won't honor your request, consider seeking a second opinion. There are plenty of doctors happy to help with supplemental screening or who encourage it.

KEEP IN MIND

You'll probably face a few important genomic decisions on your path to having your new baby. Along the way, these key points can help you make the right decision for you and your growing family.

You can undergo carrier testing for yourself, even before you are pregnant, to see if you carry a potentially risky gene that could be passed on to your baby. If you are pregnant, carrier testing poses virtually no risk to your developing baby.

If you choose to become pregnant through *in vitro* fertilization, you may have the option of having your embryos genetically analyzed before they are selected for implantation. Most doctors and fertility clinics offer this type of screening, called PGD, for families with a known history of genetic illness. Only a few offer PGD to families interested in PGD solely for the purpose of choosing the gender of their next baby, as this use of PGD is extremely controversial.

Once you are pregnant, you have a wide range of options for seeing if your developing baby carries certain genetic disorders. Some of these options, involving ultrasound scans or maternal blood tests, are less invasive, but also less conclusive. More definitive tests, such as amniocentesis, carry more risk of complications or miscarriage. These risks, while low, are worth discussing with your doctor or genetic counselor.

After birth, your baby will be tested for a series of genetic metabolic disorders. Some states, however, offer this newborn screening in much more comprehensive forms. Ask your doctor about testing options in your state, and consider supplemental screening if your state's testing is limited.

In every step of your pregnancy, these genomic testing options are almost certain to raise complicated questions about ethics and risk. While your doctors, genetic counselors, family, and friends will all have strong opinions on genetic testing and your developing baby, only you can decide what is right for you. Your genetic counselor can help you understand all the potential effects of your testing decisions as you pick the most appropriate path for you and your family.

Your baby's newborn screening test shortly after birth is likely just the first in a lifelong road to using your family's genes for better health. In looking for gene problems related to nutrition, for example, newborn screening offers your first glimpse of how your baby's genes interact with the food she eats. Over time, you'll be able to make more and more of your meals with your daughter's genes in mind. Chapter 4 looks at this growing understanding of how food works—or doesn't work—with your genes next.

CHAPTER FOUR

You Are What You Eat: Your Genes and Your Diet

Along the southern edge of Phoenix sits a stretch of Arizona desert marked by scattered clusters of cinder-block houses, three casinos, and two kidney dialysis clinics. The land belongs to the Pima Indians of the Gila River Indian Community, providing more than 10,000 tribal members a place to call home. The gambling palaces, an economic lifeline for the reservation, bring in real money for the first time in the tribe's history. And that cash helps pay for another feature of modern tribal life—the dialysis clinics and other health care offered on the reservation to combat the effects of diabetes.

Diabetes may have become commonplace in sedentary, junk food-munching America, but the condition hits Native American communities harder than any other.

Diabetes is twice as prevalent among Native Americans as it is among Caucasians, according to federal health statistics. In some tribes, more than a third of the population is diabetic. The Pima have the world's highest rate of diabetes, with the condition affecting up to 50 percent of the tribe at times. That's in comparison to a Type 2 diabetes rate of 7 percent among the rest of the United States population.

If you look in kitchens on the Pima reservation, and compare what you find to what the Pimas' ancestors ate, you might see part of the reason why tribal diabetes rates jumped so high. With the loss of traditional tribal lands and cultures, the typical Native American diet has changed rapidly in just a few generations, shifting from game and fresh produce to the flour, sugar, and fatty foods now more common in the American diet.

A diet heavy in those options would add up to increased diabetes risk in just about anyone. But something in the genes of many Native Americans appears to worsen the problem. Researchers with the National Institutes of Health have studied the health of the Pima tribe for decades, and more recently they began looking at the community's genes alongside its diet. Those studies uncovered genetic features linked to an increased susceptibility to diabetes, such as a slower metabolism and a tendency to hoard glucose, the main sugar the body uses as fuel. New studies on different reservations are trying to determine how widely other Indian tribes share these gene variants. Many gene scientists now speculate that such gene variations, mixed with a starchy, fatty diet, easily spin into an epidemic of diabetes.

In short, Native American food choices changed abruptly, but Native American DNA did not. Replace venison and corn with fat and flour, and the Indian diet may no longer be in sync with the genomic instruction manual for the Indian body.

These findings are now being used to help combat diabetes on reservations around the country. But they also extend far beyond the Pimas' tribal lands, reflecting how genomics is slowly reinventing the science of good nutrition. Scientists are increasingly able to tie one of life's essentials—your food—to the code that builds you, revealing just how much truth the adage "you are what you eat" really holds.

This new field, called nutrigenomics, examines how your food works with your genomic operating instructions. In some cases, nutrigenomics simply confirms the basics of proven nutrition—we really do, for example, need to eat our vegetables for the gene-enhancing vitamins they contain. But in many other cases, nutritional needs may be as individual as your genome. Just as the effects of a drug may differ from person to person, so may one person's ideal meal be a bad match for someone else. Nutrigenomics is helping to answer why one person's good diet advice is another's ticket to bad skin or an extra 10 pounds. Even more importantly, nutrigenomics increasingly offers insights into a range of health problems, from the current epidemics of diabetes and obesity to the digestive damage caused by celiac disease. Genes and food also play strong roles in heart disease, a condition covered in detail in Chapter 6.

This chapter covers the major components of nutrigenomics, and show how this emerging science is driving our understanding of food and health. We also review a few of the more common conditions already linked to genes and diet. In revealing the clear connections between genes, diet, and health, these conditions serve as early indicators of the promise of nutrigenomics.

Along the way, we also talk about limits that are important in helping you make the most of your genes and your food. Nutrigenomics is a new, and often uncertain, field of science. Hundreds of genes, for example, have already been associated with common conditions such as obesity, but no one is exactly sure how they all work together. This means that clear answers to questions about what foods best match your genes aren't always available—yet. We show you how to watch for nutrigenomic products and tests that may over-promise and under-deliver. In some cases, nutrigenomic innovations offer worthwhile insights. But in others, you may encounter little more than a hefty helping of hype.

Let's start by looking at the backbone of nutrigenomics—how your DNA and your diet interact.

YOUR DIET AND YOUR DNA

Since your genome carries your body's basic operating instructions, and your diet provides the fuel that keeps your body running, these two components must work together. Scientists have already learned that

Nutrigenetic Testing Has Exciting Potential, but For Now Your Dietician's Advice is More Useful

Susan, who had a daughter with PKU, called me one day with questions about genes and diet that had me stumped. I immediately called Debra, our metabolic clinic dietitian. Typically, parents of children with conditions like PKU are extremely aware of issues regarding food, genes, and general health, but sometimes a parent calls looking for cutting-edge opportunities that send us researching for answers, and Debra and I team up to respond.

Susan was visiting family in Minnesota recently and was intrigued by a genetic assessment kit she found in the vitamin aisle of a local grocery store. It turns out that Minnesota has been the testing ground for a new genetic test product and she wanted to know more. How fabulous—a chance to send a cheek swab with some DNA as well as diet and lifestyle information to a company that would provide information about her heart and bone health, her insulin resistance and her antioxidant status. Susan jumped at the opportunity to find out even more about food, genes, and general health.

Susan used the kit, but the report she received back after sending in her swab for testing was long and not easy to interpret. There was a fancy graph with X and Y axes, but they weren't even labeled! It seemed that most of the personalized advice in the report was the general information she had heard for years from her mom—eat your fruits and vegetables, don't smoke, and exercise. It didn't take into account any of her family health history or personal medical history, so although she was expecting information about her diabetic risks, that wasn't included. And the really annoying part is that she was advised to add a lot of supplements to her relatively well-balanced diet. Susan was frustrated that this didn't live up to the exciting promise she had expected. After reviewing the report, Debra and I could understand why.

Bottom Line: As a genetic counselor, I invite my patients to ask lots of questions about current nutrigenetic testing claims. There is exciting potential in this new field that associates genetic markers with common health conditions and provides useful advice for using everyday foods to promote health and prevent disease. However, the existing products are confusing and not that helpful, even for people like Susan, who are early adopters of new alternative health products. The reason is that there are scant data about many of these genetic markers and even less on how they interact with each other or with the many and different foods you eat. It would be a shame if the interested consumers ignore future discoveries because of the immature science that is currently being marketed.

Someday soon, the association between genetic information and diet will be clearer for people in the general population. But for now, a consult with a qualified dietician will provide advice that is likely more useful than the nutrigenetic tests for using your genetic make-up to influence the way you eat.

many diet-related physical functions, such as your ability to digest milk and dairy products, start in the genes. In some cases, such as with the Pima Indians, these interactions can flare into serious long-term health problems, such as diabetes or high cholesterol.

Scientists are also looking beyond specific, well-known food-related diseases such as obesity or diabetes. Nutrigenomics assumes, at its broadest level, that growing genomic knowledge can help you build a better grocery list. By studying how your genes interact with your food, this field of research hopes to help you achieve optimum overall health. You might, over time, be able to match your diet with the specific workings of your individual genome, and focus on which foods provide your body's optimum fuel. Some nutrigenomic scientists theorize that new types of functional foods with demonstrated health claims could someday arise from nutrigenomic research. These foods would, in theory, help certain genes or sections of your genome work more efficiently and boost your health.

A more DNA-linked diet starts with an understanding of how individual nutrients, the building blocks of nutrition, work with DNA. Once it enters your body, your food breaks down into basic components in your digestive system and blood stream. If you eat a plate of pasta for lunch, for example, your body dissolves the meal into its component molecules of fats, proteins, and sugars. These molecules interact with the cells of your body—including the DNA they hold—sometimes affecting how your genome does its job. In other cases, it's your DNA that takes action on your food, issuing instructions for how certain nutrients should be handled. Some nutrients are immediately put to good use, such as a vitamin that boosts your immune system when you have a cold. Other nutrients, such as extra fats, might be unnecessary at that time, and packed into fat cells for long-term storage.

These interactions form the foundation of several key areas of nutrigenomic research:

- The first examines the general ways in which DNA and diet interact to shape human health. As revealed by the blend of lifestyle and genetic factors that contribute to Type 2 diabetes, diet is clearly an important risk factor for a number of DNA-linked conditions.
- The second looks at how each person's individual genetic make-up relates differently to food. While certain foods increase the risk of diabetes in general, for example, some people's genes clearly put them more at risk than others.
- The third studies food's power to affect genes, and whether specially tailored diets have the potential to prevent, ease, or even cure some diseases.

Through a sharper understanding of nutrition and genes, nutrigenomic researchers hope to eventually help people to stay healthier by matching their diet to their DNA. Some even envision individual eating plans based on each person's genes.

You can't build your own fully personalized menu for health just yet. But recent changes in nutritional recommendations, combined with some essentials of personalized medicine, are giving you some new options for picking foods that suit you best. As with every other aspect of your health, DNA research is shaking apart broad recommendations about what *everyone* should do, letting you instead think about what *you* should do.

STARTING A "DNA DIET"

Until the emergence of DNA-based nutritional research, eating rarely got truly individualized scrutiny. We are all used to hearing the same dietary advice—eating vegetables and drinking milk is good for you, lots of fat is bad, refined sugar rots your teeth.

Gene research is revealing plenty of exceptions to these general rules. Dairy products may be healthful source of calcium—unless you suffer from lactose intolerance, a common condition now linked to a gene variant. Some people, their genes wired for cholesterol trouble, suffer more from

IT'S YOUR CHOICE

Can Nutrigenomics Help You Feed Your Family?

If you have a family, mealtime means at least a few mouths to feed. You probably often find yourself choosing and cooking meals not only for yourself, but also for your spouse, your children, or older relatives who live with you. That can make eating with genes in mind more complicated, as you'll find yourself making gene-related decisions on behalf of others as well as yourself. If you are considering the most beneficial ways to balance your family's genes and food, here are some points to keep in mind:

- Be wary of commercial genetic tests that claim to provide easy answers about DNA and diet, especially when it comes to your children. Independent studies have found that many of these tests are unproven and unreliable. And these tests may not take the special nutritional needs of growing children into account. Doctors advise against them.
- Steer clear of commercial vitamin and supplement blends that claim to be matched to your family's genes. An independent study found that the contents of these blends could pose health risks of their own. This is especially true for young children, who may be more sensitive to high levels of certain substances.
- Your family medical history is the best place to start tracking any genetic food-related troubles that run in your bloodline. If your family history reveals such a problem, talk to your family doctor or nutritionist about crafting an appropriate eating plan.
- Remember, everyone's genome is unique. Even your children, who inherited their genes from you and your spouse, aren't carbon copies of each other or the two of you. There may be no one-menu-for-all approach that works for your entire family.
- If you aren't yet sure how to balance your family's genes and food, rest assured you can still fall back on the basics of good nutrition for now. Most current nutritional advice, while very broad, is based on good science that can guide you while the science of nutrigenomics grows.

Feeding your family is a big responsibility. By starting from a foundation of good basic nutrition, you'll be able to make healthful choices while nutrigenomics develops the tools to one day help reshape the contents of your kitchen.

the effects of high levels of saturated fat in their diet. Sugar is bad for anyone's teeth, but in people at risk for diabetes, sugars must be watched closely to prevent serious health problems that go beyond cavities.

Such findings raise important questions about the dietary rules most of us try to live by. For decades, food guidelines in the United States applied to everyone equally, usually expressed in one format for all—the food pyramid. This icon of healthful eating spelled out which types of food, such as saturated fats and refined sugars, should be consumed in smaller amounts and which, such as fruits and vegetables, should be a large part of a sound diet. The traditional food pyramid, developed by the U.S. Department of Agriculture (USDA), assumed that when it comes to a good diet, we are all pretty much the same. This approach said a great deal about good nutrition for the population as a whole. It said very little about what's best for you individually.

But in 2005, the USDA took steps to make its recommendations a bit more specific, changing its pyramid for all to a series of pyramids for different groups, based on age, gender, and exercise level. Using a Web-based nutrition calculator, found at www.mypyramid.gov, you can enter your personal information and receive nutrition recommendations built for your group. When it comes to drinking milk, for example, the new pyramid says a five-year-old girl who gets less than 30 minutes of exercise a day should drink 2 cups of milk a day. A much larger, much older 30-year-old man who works out for up to an hour a day, on the other hand, is urged to drink 3 cups of milk.

It's true that these dietary guidelines still remain very broad. They assume, for example, that all 30-year-old men who spend an hour a day at the gym benefit from basically the same diet, regardless of factors such as ethnic background or family medical history. But you can combine these guidelines with one of the aids in your personalized medicine toolkit—your family medical history—to come up with a version of this new food pyramid that also reflects your DNA.

Another Approach to the Food Pyramid

The USDA has done a lot of work to promote its new, more specific food pyramids, but not all nutrition experts agree with how they work. At the Harvard School of Public Health, for example, nutrition experts fault the revised guidelines for allowing too many refined carbohydrates and not offering alternatives to dairy products. Unlike the USDA, Harvard's experts note that millions of Americans have trouble digesting milk and dairy products, often for genetic reasons covered later in this chapter. Harvard put together a food pyramid that offers a different approach from the USDA. You can review it at www.hsph.harvard.edu/nutritionsource/pyramids.html. If something in your genetic profile or family history leaves you uncomfortable with some of the suggestions in the USDA pyramids, these guidelines might be a better fit for you.

If you are the 30-year-old man described above, for example, the recommendations make it clear that you need the protein and calcium found in milk. But perhaps your own health experiences, along with your family medical history, also show a tendency toward lactose intolerance. In that case, getting protein and calcium from milk might not be your best option. But you could get your protein from other foods, such as fish or meat, and take calcium supplements. Factoring in your family history makes your food pyramid that much more personal. You can also talk to your doctor or nutritionist about your family history, and seek their advice on what your genetic legacy says about your diet.

If you want to start eating with your genes in mind, however, it's also important to remember that you'll need to be extra savvy. While some diet-related genes are well known, many others are still being researched, including DNA links to weight gain, cholesterol trouble, and the immune system responses tied to food allergies. Genes and weight concerns are covered later in this chapter. Cholesterol gets more discussion in Chapter 6, and more information on genes and allergies is found in Chapter 9.

Given all the questions scientists still need to answer about genes and diet, it's worth being cautious of commercial genetic tests that claim they can answer complicated questions about your genes and nutrition easily. A recent Congressional study of nutrigenomic tests sold online, for example, found that some of these tests "mislead consumers by making predictions that are medically unproven and so ambiguous that they do not provide meaningful information."

Products such as personalized vitamins or other expensive nutritional supplements supposedly tailored to your genes also deserve a healthy dose of skepticism. These vitamin offers usually start with a genetic test that claims to analyze your genes for important food-related factors. The company selling the test then offers to make you batches of vitamins specially tailored to your genome. But since so many key food-related genes and their effects aren't fully understood, these expensive vitamin packages are probably of little value. The same Congressional study found that one set of these so-called personalized supplements would cost about $1,200 a year, but the ingredients in that blend of supplements matched those of grocery store vitamins and supplements costing about $35 a year. Until our understanding of genes and nutrition improves, genomic experts agree that you are better off trusting your common sense and family history over unproven nutrigenomic vitamins and supplements.

You can also boost your understanding of your genes and your diet by learning more about conditions where the link between genes and food is already clear. Some of these conditions may run in your family. Others may be health concerns you've heard about from friends or through news reports. Together, they reveal a glimpse of the future of DNA and diet, when what you eat will be tied to who you are.

LACTOSE INTOLERANCE

Lactose intolerance is the inability to digest lactose, a naturally occurring sugar found in milk and many dairy products. It is caused by a deficiency of lactase, an enzyme that digests milk sugar.

Newborn babies require milk to thrive, and their bodies normally produce lactase, although amounts of this enzyme can vary widely from person to person. But in the majority of the world's population, production of this enzyme starts to decline later in childhood and through early adulthood. This lactase decline is so common worldwide that in many places, it's considered normal—and the lifelong milk drinkers stand out as unusual. In the United States, for example, scientific papers talk about lactose intolerance, while scientists in Asian countries refer to the less common version of milk digestion as lactose tolerance.

Few children whose bodies gradually stop making lactase ever show symptoms of lactose intolerance before the age of six. But by the age of 20, many Americans show symptoms of lactose intolerance, and at least 75 percent of the world's people experience age-related lactase decline. Lactose intolerance can also appear from birth, although such congenital cases are less common.

RED FLAG!

More Problems with Nutrigenomic Tests

The Congressional inquiry into commercial nutrigenomic tests found that, in numerous cases, these services either mislead consumers or have the potential to harm someone's health. Here are three major concerns highlighted in the study:

- The tests all predicted that the test subjects were at risk for developing a range of health problems, including cancer, osteoporosis, and high blood pressure, even though, as the investigation noted, "the medical predictions in the test results cannot be medically proven at this time."
- Some of the personalized vitamins and supplements recommended by the companies could actually be harmful. One company, for example, recommended an herbal supplement that can trigger adverse reactions if taken with some prescription medication. While there's a chance of harmful interactions with any supplement, experts who helped with the report said this particular blend posed especially noteworthy risks.
- Many of the health recommendations offered with genetic test results seemed to be grounded more in common sense than any concrete knowledge of the test subject's genome. People who said they'd never smoked, for example, received recommendations to continue to avoid smoking.

The bottom line, investigators said, is that many nutrigenomic tests appear to be nothing more than an expensive waste of time and money. Some Congressional lawmakers are considering tougher regulation of commercial genetic tests.

Without sufficient lactase in the digestive system, lactose travels through the digestive tract without breaking down. The result, simply put, is gut trouble. Symptoms include abdominal bloating, gas, nausea, diarrhea, and cramps.

Lactose intolerance is rarely serious, with digestive discomfort the most common problem. In severe cases, some malnutrition may result if symptoms persist for long periods of time, impeding appetite.

How genes are involved

The gene for lactase production, as well as at least three variants that appear to be connected to lactose intolerance, have been mapped to a particular section of Chromosome 2. These genes are considered responsible for rare cases in which babies are lactose intolerant from birth, as well as the much more common age-related form of the condition.

Genetic testing for lactose intolerance

Most common tests for lactose intolerance are not gene-based. A doctor may simply tell you to avoid dairy products and see if your symptoms disappear. Other testing methods involve a blood sugar analysis, a test

Milk Drinkers are Mutants

Drink milk, standard diet advice says. You can't find a better source of bone-building calcium.

But for a majority of the world's people—including as many as 50 million Americans—that recommendation often spells more digestion trouble than good nutrition. Many people of African-American, Asian-American, and Latino descent have long complained that following advice to drink milk gives them digestive upset. But nutrition guidelines didn't budge. If people just tried drinking more milk, some nutritionists suggested, their digestive systems might adjust.

Now, gene research has turned that advice upside-down. People who drink milk and enjoy dairy products throughout their entire lives are the abnormal ones, beneficiaries of a gene mutation. Adults who look askance at a bowl of ice cream reflect the human genomic norm.

Lactose intolerance affects more than 75 percent of the world's people, especially those who aren't descended from northern Europeans. Gene researchers have learned that most people with northern European ancestry carry a genetic mutation on Chromosome 2 that leaves milk digestion switched on throughout their lives. This mutation can also easily override its dairy-adverse variant, meaning that many people of mixed ancestry have also picked up the ability to digest milk as adults.

Americans of northern European descent first developed many of the nutrition guidelines in this country, including the focus on milk. As the country grows more diverse, however, many nutritionists and doctors are learning to shift their dietary advice for people from other backgrounds.

that measures the amount of hydrogen in your breath (raised levels of hydrogen indicate improper digestion of lactose), and a stool-sample test.

Several companies now also offer commercial genetic tests for adult-onset lactase decline. Most of these deliver results by looking at a SNP related to lactase production.

In some situations, however, this test may not provide better answers than regular types of diagnosis. Many doctors say they are reluctant to order the gene test for adult-onset decline in lactose production, citing the cost—usually in the hundreds of dollars—and lack of insurance coverage. Also, a genetic test result alone does not tell you if you have an active case of lactose intolerance. You'll need to compare your genetic results along-side any current symptoms and traditional forms of diagnosis.

Special considerations for lactose intolerance

Not all lactose intolerance is caused by congenital or long-term lactase deficiency. Short-term illnesses, such as gastroenteritis, or other long-term digestive inflammation, such as that caused by celiac disease, can also lead to trouble digesting lactase.

How you can treat lactose intolerance

The most common and effective treatment simply removes dairy products and other foods containing lactose from the diet. After dropping dairy products, lactose intolerance sufferers are usually encouraged to look for other sources of calcium, such as supplements. Care must also be taken in choosing processed foods, as many contain lactose.

In many areas, grocery stores sell lactose-free milk and other lactose-free dairy products. Lactase enzymes can also be added to milk or taken in supplement form.

CELIAC DISEASE

Celiac disease (also called celiac sprue) is an autoimmune disorder triggered by exposure to gluten, a common component in grains such as wheat, rye, and barley. In people with celiac disease, gluten triggers an immune response that attacks and damages the lining of the small intestine. Small finger-like projections of tissue, called villi, shape this lining and absorb nutrients. In people with celiac disease, the immune reaction to gluten flattens and distorts these villi, diminishing the ability to absorb nutrients from food.

Once thought rare, celiac disease actually appears to affect as many as 1 in 133 Americans, according to a major study published in 2003 in the journal *Archives of Internal Medicine*. Women and people of Caucasian and European ancestry develop the disease most often. For reasons not yet understood, the disease can develop at any point in life, from infancy to late adulthood.

The symptoms of celiac disease often vary widely from person to person. Many develop painful abdominal bloating, while others eventually develop clear signs of malnutrition, such as anemia or weight loss. Nausea, vomiting, and diarrhea are also common symptoms. Because of the variability of symptoms, the disease can be difficult to diagnose and is often mistaken for other digestive disorders.

If left untreated, serious health problems can result, including anemia, skin disorders, delayed or limited growth in children, and bone disease.

How genes are involved

Doctors have long known that a family history of celiac disease increases a person's risk of developing the condition. First-degree relatives of a celiac patient (parents, children, siblings) have a 1 in 22 chance of developing celiac disease in their lifetimes, according to the 2003 celiac disease study.

More recently, researchers linked two genes, *HLA-DQ2* and *HLA-DQ8* on Chromosome 6, to celiac disease. Doctors now say celiac-related variants of these genes are necessary for the disease to develop. Scientists suspect that other genes also play a role, but have not yet uncovered them.

Genetic testing for celiac disease

Several commercial gene tests are now available for genetic variants related to celiac disease. Most look for alleles or SNPs related to *HLA-DQ2* and/or *HLA-DQ8* gene variants linked to the condition.

More routine diagnostic tests include blood tests that measure celiac-related antibodies and the immune system's response to gluten in food. Doctors sometimes consider an intestinal biopsy to check for tissue damage as the most conclusive way to diagnose the condition.

The decision to take a genetic test related to celiac should be considered carefully. These forms of testing, using a saliva or blood sample, are less invasive than a procedure such an intestinal biopsy. But *HLA-DQ2* and *HLA-DQ8* tests are not definitive. They work best at ruling out celiac—if a person does not have these gene variants, there is almost no chance they will ever develop celiac disease. If one or both of the genes are

Did You Know?

Hidden ingredients in packaged and processed foods make it difficult for people with celiac disease to reach for snacks or enjoy restaurant meals. Nutrition experts say the following ingredients, a common sight on many food labels, usually mean that a grain containing gluten probably lurks in the food:

- Stabilizer
- Starch
- Flavoring
- Emulsifier
- Hydrolyzed plant protein

If you have celiac disease or are concerned about gluten in your diet, doctors recommend avoiding any food you're unsure of. Instead, seek out gluten-free products and recipes. You can find plenty of cookbooks for gluten-free dishes, and people with celiac disease can now also find gluten-free brownies, pasta, and even pizza.

present, a person is at elevated risk, but is not certain to develop celiac disease. If the test reveals these gene variants, regular monitoring for celiac disease or further testing is recommended.

Special considerations for celiac disease

Celiac disease can be extremely difficult to diagnose, and misdiagnosis is common. Many people suffer from symptoms for years as a result. If celiac disease is suspected, a thorough range of tests is the best way to detect the condition. Relatives of people who have been diagnosed with celiac disease should undergo regular monitoring for signs of the condition.

How you can treat celiac disease

No cure is yet available, but people with celiac disease can stop and even reverse intestinal tissue damage by removing gluten from their diet. The widespread presence of gluten in regular foods, however, makes avoiding it a challenge. People with celiac disease must refrain from common gluten foods such as regular wheat-based bread, pasta, or cookies baked with wheat flour, as well as many processed and restaurant foods such as soy sauce and commercially prepared French fries. Most processed foods include grain-based fillers or flavorings that include gluten.

Researchers hope to develop a medicine or supplement that would allow people with celiac disease to tolerate gluten, but none are yet available.

OBESITY

In simple terms, being obese means being very overweight. Obesity determinations are usually made by using a person's height and weight to calculate a figure called the body mass index, or BMI, tied to a person's amount of body fat. You can calculate your own BMI by dividing your weight in pounds by the square of your height in inches, and then multiply that result by 703. In adults, a BMI of 25 or higher means you are overweight, and a BMI of 30 or higher is considered obese, according to the federal Centers for Disease Control and Prevention. Health experts also increasingly recommend paying attention to the size of your waist, as abdominal fat has been linked to a greater risk of health problems. The International Diabetes Federation, for example, recommends a waist circumference of less than 37 inches for men, and less than 31.5 inches for women.

But obesity is rarely as simple as doing a little math or reaching for the tape measure. Rates of obesity are rising in the United States and around the world—as of the mid-2000s, for example, federal health officials said almost 25 percent of all Americans were obese. As any obese person trying to lose weight will say, the condition proves extremely challenging to reverse. Scientists say a variety of factors—including our increasingly sedentary lifestyles, diets containing larger portions of high-sugar, high-fat processed foods, and metabolic responses to these foods that trigger excessive weight gain—all help drive up rates of obesity.

Obesity increases a person's risk of disease and death due to diabetes, stroke, heart disease, high blood pressure, and kidney disorders. Obesity may also increase the risk for some types of cancer, and can also cause joint pain, mobility problems, and arthritis.

How genes are involved

In a few cases, obesity can be directly pinned on a gene. Some rare developmental disorders, such as a condition called Prader-Willi syndrome, can be clearly linked to genes that fuel excessive weight gain.

Genomic science has revealed that more common forms of obesity are much more complex. So far, more than 300 genomic factors have been linked to obesity. Different gene variants may also trigger a greater likelihood of obesity in different people. And in virtually all people, a mix of genes may work alongside diet and exercise choices to encourage excessive weight gain.

For example, scientists are studying a gene called *GAD2*, which appears to be strongly associated with obesity. *GAD2* helps stimulate the desire to eat. One variation of the gene appears to increase the risk of obesity, while another appears to lower it. More recently, an American-led research team located a section of Chromosome 2 that appears to hold a very common stretch of DNA related to obesity. This part of Chromosome 2 holds genes related to fat metabolism, and certain variations in one or more of these genes may make a person more prone to storing fat.

But could all cases of obesity be linked to *GAD2* or Chromosome 2? No, researchers say. It is unlikely that DNA will ever be singled out as the sole cause of most common cases of obesity.

The Obesity Gene

Gene experts gave up looking for one primary genetic culprit to blame for our expanding waistlines long ago. While news of the discovery of a particular gene related to obesity often makes headlines, it's far more likely that many genes contribute to our expanding waistlines. These genes are being catalogued by a scientific project known as the Obesity Gene Map. Updated every year, the map shows hundreds of genes either directly or indirectly linked to obesity. Most genes on the map fall into one of three categories—those that influence your appetite, those that control your metabolism, and those that shape how your body stores fat.

Scientists hope that by gathering and sharing information on all these genes in one place, they'll be able to come up with better genomic explanations for what drives obesity. Just as controlling your weight means balancing your genes and your lifestyle, understanding your genomic risks for obesity means knowing how hundreds of your genes work together.

Genetic testing for obesity

Several companies now offer genetic tests related to obesity. Most of these focus on SNPs showing some linkage to excess weight, and are usually included in a group of other genetic results that costs at least several hundred dollars.

It is important to remember, though, that the results of these tests aren't definitive. The genetic variants they analyze may contribute to weight gain, but they don't cause it on their own. Genetic results can't guarantee you will become obese, or tell you how to take the weight off if you are. They can, however, indicate if you are at increased risk, information that might help you focus your eating and exercise habits on controlling weight gain.

Special considerations for obesity

A genetic tendency towards of obesity is not destiny—or an excuse. While family history can indicate increased risk, it also points out the need for preventive measures. Even if your DNA is working against you, doctors stress that you can still take important nutrition and fitness steps to reduce your risk of obesity and protect your health.

How you can treat obesity

Most treatments begin with a controlled, lower-calorie diet and stepped-up exercise routine. Psychological support through weight-loss groups may also help. If those measures fail, more drastic weight controls, such as bariatric surgery to reduce the size of a person's stomach and limit food intake, may also be considered, but usually only if your weight exceeds 300 pounds. Remember that even if your DNA puts you at increased risk for obesity, your diet and lifestyle also have a lot to say about your weight.

DIABETES

Diabetes is a chronic condition marked by difficulties metabolizing glucose, a common sugar, resulting in consistently high blood sugar levels. The disorder can be caused by the body producing too little insulin, a hormone that regulates blood sugar, resistance to insulin, or both. Left unchecked, high blood sugar levels can trigger potentially dangerous health problems, including long-term tissue damage, blindness, and seizures.

Diabetes is one of the most common health problems in the United States, with rates rising in this country and worldwide, according to the National Institutes of Health. More than 20 million Americans had diabetes as of 2005, according to agency calculations.

There are three major forms of the disease:

- **Juvenile diabetes, also called type 1.** Usually diagnosed in childhood, this form of diabetes typically requires frequent injections of insulin to control blood sugar.
- **Adult-onset diabetes, also called type 2.** This is the most common form of diabetes, representing about 90 percent of all cases. Decades of research have linked type 2 diabetes to poor diet, obesity, and little exercise. In about five percent of adult-onset diabetes cases, certain rare gene variants play a strong role. In other people, more common but less powerful gene variants may also contribute to the condition.
- **Gestational diabetes.** This condition refers to high blood sugar levels that arise in some women during pregnancy. It often subsides after pregnancy, but women with gestational diabetes are at increased risk of developing type 2 diabetes later in life. If you are an expectant mother, several factors put you at greater risk for gestational diabetes, including African or Hispanic ancestry, obesity, having a previous baby who weighed more than 9 pounds, or a previous case of gestational diabetes.

A Gene Variant's Role in Insulin Resistance

Eager to bring advanced genomic tools into the fight against diabetes, a team of scientists and doctors in France and the United States has uncovered how one gene disables some peoples' ability to maintain healthy blood sugar levels.

Their search started with a protein called PC-1. People with diabetes carry unusually high levels of this protein in their blood. PC-1 deactivates another important protein, called the insulin receptor. Insulin, a hormone in your body, is key to regulating the level of sugar in your blood. If PC-1 deactivates your insulin receptors, your body can't readily keep your blood sugar under control. This is called insulin resistance syndrome, and it is a major factor in many cases of type 2 diabetes and obesity, affecting about 50 million Americans and an equal number of people in Europe. It doubles a person's risk of heart attack or stroke, and triples their risk of dying early from either cause.

The team of scientists decided to find out why people with diabetes carried so much PC-1. Since proteins arise from genes, they started studying the gene that carries the instructions for making PC-1. The international team of scientists signed up 3,000 people in France, and began an extensive study of variations in their *PC-1* genes, located on Chromosome 6. They found that a common variant of the *PC-1* gene, combined with a few other small changes on the gene, increases PC-1 production and is closely linked with insulin resistance, type 2 diabetes, and obesity.

The team released its findings in 2005, and immediately began thinking about a new medical target. Rather than just managing diabetes, the findings point to potential drugs to restore the body's ability to respond to insulin. Many of the same researchers are now studying what therapies might be developed to counteract the problem of PC-1, and perhaps help stem the rise of this form of insulin resistance and diabetes.

Symptoms for both type 1 and type 2 diabetes include frequent thirst, increased urination, blurred vision, and fatigue. Type 1 patients may also suffer weight loss, nausea, and vomiting.

How genes are involved

Some well-known risk factors for diabetes strongly indicate a genetic link. If diabetes runs in your family, for example, you are also at higher risk. The condition arises more frequently in some population groups, including Native Americans, African-Americans, and Latinos.

Recent research has further pinpointed more than 200 gene variants that appear to be linked to diabetes. A mutation on a gene called *SUMO-4*, for example, has been linked to juvenile diabetes. The mutation appears more frequently in people with type 1 diabetes, and increases the activity of a protein related to an autoimmune response that underlies this type of diabetes. In the case of type 2 diabetes, researchers have found a gene on Chromosome 20 called *PTPN1* that may be linked to as many as 20 percent of adult-onset cases. This gene makes a protein that represses the body's insulin response.

About five percent of adults with type 2 diabetes can pin their condition directly to certain genes. People with this form of diabetes, called Mature-Onset Diabetes of the Young, or MODY, have any one of at least six different gene mutations that limit their body's ability to release insulin. They often develop diabetes in their late teens or 20s, and tend not to share common risk factors for type 2 diabetes, such as being overweight.

No one gene or set of genes, however, has been named as the definitive cause of most cases of diabetes. Diabetes is a complex condition, likely arising from multiple gene variants and influenced by your diet, exercise, and other lifestyle choices. Many gene variants may simply increase your risk of diabetes, rather than directly cause it.

Genetic testing for diabetes

Your family history is the easiest place to start looking for any inherited risk. But keep in mind that with this condition, family history isn't always definitive. A family history free of diabetes does not mean you will never develop the disease. And if diabetes does run in your family, good preventive health measures can lower your risk.

Several companies now offer genetic testing that analyzes SNPs related to type 2 diabetes risk. If you are considering such a test, however, keep in mind that the results are not conclusive. Increased genetic risk does not guarantee you will develop the condition. And these tests may not analyze all DNA linked to diabetes. If such a test does find that you are at increased risk, however, you may find the knowledge helpful in guiding your eating, exercise, and other prevention choices.

If your doctor suspects you have MODY, however, more conclusive testing is available. Your doctor has the option of ordering a genetic test that looks for MODY-related mutations. It's also important to keep in mind that since MODY mutations are responsible for only a small fraction of diabetes cases, a negative MODY test result does not mean that you don't have diabetes, and can't eliminate your diabetes risk.

Special considerations for diabetes

Your family history or genetic risk of diabetes can indicate whether or not you are likely to develop the condition. But many factors within your control, such as diet and exercise, remain very important. If you know you have a family history or genetic tendency toward diabetes, a health care plan involving specific diet and exercise regimens can help lower your chances of developing the condition.

How you can treat diabetes

There is no cure for types 1 and 2 diabetes. Patients must adopt a life-long regimen of monitoring their diet and blood sugar levels. Some type 2 patients can control their diabetes through diet and exercise. For other type 2 patients and almost all type 1 patients, drugs and/or insulin injections are usually required to keep blood sugar levels under control.

PHENYLKETONURIA

Phenylketonuria (PKU) is a nutritional disorder that strikes babies at birth. Babies born with PKU have two abnormal copies of the PKU gene, found on Chromosome 12. This mutation leaves them unable to properly process phenylalanine, an amino acid found in high-protein foods such as milk, meat, and fish. Phenylalanine builds up to dangerous levels in their bodies, causing damage to the brain and central nervous system. If left unchecked, PKU leads to serious developmental disabilities by a child's first birthday.

PKU is relatively rare, occurring in about 1 in every 10,000 to 20,000 births. It is the most common of a large series of disorders known as inborn errors of metabolism. Many states now test newborn babies for PKU and similar metabolic disorders. (For more information on newborn screening, see Chapter 3.)

How genes are involved

PKU arises from a mutation on alleles for the gene for phenylalanine hydroxylase, or *PAH*. The mutations render the gene inactive or less efficient than normal. The condition is recessive, meaning that a person must inherit two copies of a related mutation to develop PKU. A person with only one copy is considered a carrier, who can pass on the mutation but will not develop the disorder. Two carrier parents have a 25 percent chance with each pregnancy of having a child with PKU. The disease is found worldwide, but is most common among Caucasians and Asians.

Genetic testing for PKU

Though gene testing can detect PKU mutations, this is not the most common form of screening. In every state, newborn babies now undergo a simple blood test for PKU and other inborn errors of metabolism. The test detects substances in the blood related to PKU, rather than screening for PKU genes. (For more information on newborn screening, see Chapter 3.)

If PKU is diagnosed through this newborn blood test, further testing may include an injection of phenylalanine to see how your baby's body processes the amino acid. Gene screening may be recommended to look for the PKU mutation. Expectant parents with a history of PKU in their family should ask their doctor for carrier screening to help gauge any risks to their babies. Prenatal testing, usually conducted through amniocentesis, is available when a developing fetus is considered at risk of PKU. (For more information on prenatal testing, see Chapter 3).

Special considerations for PKU

People with any family history of PKU should consider carrier testing if planning a family. And an unusual phenomenon has occurred as new generations of women with PKU have begun having babies. Although the majority of those babies do not have PKU, they spend the first nine months of their lives in a pheylalanine-enriched environment *in utero*. Subsequently, these children have concerns that may include unusual facial features, heart defects, and mental retardations and possibly fetal death. Adult women with PKU are advised to follow a low-phenylalanine diet if pregnant, as high levels of the amino acid can damage unborn babies, even if the baby has not inherited a PKU-related mutation.

How you can treat PKU

There is no cure for PKU, but the condition can be controlled, and brain damage limited or averted, by following a diet extremely low in phenylalanine, especially when a child is young. This means limiting or avoiding common protein-rich foods such as meat and eggs, as well as the common artificial sweetener NutraSweet, which contains phenylalanine. Doctors have found that if children with PKU can stick to such a diet, they have a good chance of living healthy, normal lives.

FREQUENTLY ASKED QUESTIONS ON GENES AND NUTRITION

Q. Why are there so many unanswered questions about genes and nutrition? If scientists can figure out why a rare disease is caused by a gene, why can't they understand something as routine as how my genes interact with my food?

A. It's true that your genes interact with the food you eat every single day. But this interaction is very complex, involving many genes at any one time. Rare genetic diseases, on the other hand, usually involve just one problematic gene. It's far easier to isolate one gene and its effects than many different ones. The complexity of nutrigenomic science forces researchers to go more slowly.

Q. Common diet recommendations seem so broad that I'm not sure they're meaningful. If my genes really have a big effect on my diet, why should I even pay attention to things like general dietary guidelines?

A. Broad nutritional guidelines have solid science behind them. They were developed by studying the effects of certain foods in large groups of people, and offer advice that many people find helpful. But it's also true that not every general dietary recommendation may be right for you. Take your family history into account, and talk with your doctor or nutritionist if some standard piece of nutrition advice doesn't seem to be a good fit for you.

Q. My daughter has all the symptoms of celiac disease, but no one will take us seriously. One doctor told us she might have an ulcer, but ulcer medication didn't seem to help. Another doctor asked if she might be anorexic. How can I find someone to take my questions seriously?

A. Your dilemma is one common to people with celiac disease. Many tell stories of being misdiagnosed for years before getting the help they needed. Find a celiac disease specialist who will help you understand your daughter's symptoms and order any necessary tests. The Celiac Disease Foundation, with a Web site at www.celiac.org, can help connect you with doctors and families with the condition in your area.

Q. My mom was very obese. So was my dad. Of my four brothers and sisters, only one isn't a size XXL. If fat just seems to run in our family, why should we even bother to find the right diet?

A. It's true that in some families, obesity appears to have a genetic connection. But in many families, obesity is also the result of lifestyle choices that involve large and/or unhealthy meals and sedentary lifestyles. If there is a genetic component to the obesity in your family, certain foods may increase your likelihood of gaining more weight than is healthful. You and your family may never be petite, but a healthful diet can work with your genes to help you control your weight and protect you from long-term complications of obesity, such as heart disease or diabetes. Talk to your doctor or nutritionist about developing an eating and exercise plan that helps you counteract any genetic factors that may contribute to your weight gain. And remember, your genes don't equal your fate.

Q. Both my parents had type 2 diabetes, but I seem fine. I'm not worried about me, but what about my kids?

A. When it comes to genes and diabetes, so many unknowns remain that you have good reason for both relief and concern. It's great that you've avoided diabetes, and your good health is a good sign for your children. But you may also have a more healthful lifestyle than your parents, and your children might need to consider that as they seek to prevent diabetes themselves later in their lives. Talk to your kids about their family history of diabetes. Even if you're not sure they've inherited any increased risk, their family information can help them develop a preventive health plan that helps them follow in your footsteps.

KEEP IN MIND

As you consider your own DNA diet, these key points can help you make the most of this new area of genomic health. Nutrigenomics carries a great deal of promise. But this field of science is also still very new.

You can already use one important aspect of personalized medicine—your family medical history—to make existing dietary guidelines suit you better. If your family history reveals a problem such as lactose intolerance, for example, talk to your doctor or nutritionist about how you can get the nutrition you need through other foods.

Be skeptical of commercial vitamins or supplements that claim they can match your genes. The science just isn't there to back up these tests, and currently these products are probably a waste of money.

No matter what your genes say, nutrition is one area in which your choices have a big effect. Study your family history to get a sense of your risks for conditions such as diabetes, and work with your doctor or nutritionist to develop an eating plan to help reduce your risk.

Nutrigenomic scientists hope that their work will eventually provide you even better answers for keeping yourself healthy and preventing serious illnesses such as diabetes, or even cancer. Nexrt we look more closely at cancer, and how genomic tools give you new weapons against this DNA-driven disease.

CHAPTER FIVE

YOUR GENES AND CANCER: FINDING YOUR RISKS, BOOSTING YOUR OPTIONS

In Parker Lee's genome, changes in her DNA led to a sobering diagnosis—breast cancer. But her cancerous DNA also yielded a secret that let her fight the disease, on her terms.

Parker's fight against cancer had started typically enough. She had first noticed a lump in her left breast while taking a shower at the gym and scheduled an appointment with her doctor right away. She was in her late 40s—a little young for breast cancer—and her doctor tried to reassure her that the lump probably wasn't anything serious. But Parker pushed for a thorough range of tests, which uncovered a dangerous tumor. Wanting to take no chances with her health, Parker had opted for a double mastectomy to remove the cancer and try to prevent its return.

Her tough decisions didn't end with her surgery. Happily, the cancer had not spread to her lymph nodes, and there were no obvious signs that it had invaded other parts of her body. She hoped that the mastectomy would be enough treatment. But as an extra protection against any return of breast cancer, doctors often recommend follow-up chemotherapy after the type of surgery that Parker underwent. Many women like Parker probably don't need chemotherapy, but since doctors have long been unable to tell whose tumors are more likely to recur, the powerful drugs have become standard practice in treating many breast cancers.

But Parker didn't want to follow that route. As a busy entrepreneur and mom, she was responsible for a small business and two children. She preferred to avoid further treatment if possible, especially chemotherapy and its unpleasant side effects of hair loss, nausea, and fatigue. She did a little research, and found a new test that analyzed a breast tumor's genes and might predict the chances of the cancer returning. Thanks to this genomic advance in decoding cancer, she and her doctor might just be able to clarify her prospects for another bout of breast cancer, helping Parker make her decision about chemotherapy.

After talking with her doctor—and weighing the fact that the new test might not yield a definitive answer—Parker chose to have her tumor evaluated. The genetic pattern of the tumor predicted that her cancer had a low chance of returning. After further conversations with her doctors, she decided against chemotherapy. Several years later and still cancer-free, she couldn't be happier about her decision.

"I feel lucky to have had that choice," she says. "It let me safely avoid a really tough part of cancer treatment. It let me return to my normal life sooner—and getting back to my kids and my job was the best medicine of all."

Parker's experience comes as part of some of the biggest advances in the fight against cancer in decades. New genomic tests and medicines are reinventing our options for preventing, diagnosing, and treating this difficult disease. These innovations are possible, in part, because cancer's very nature gives genomic medicine unique advantages. The disease arises when DNA becomes abnormal or damaged, triggering once-healthy cells to start growing out of control. Some people inherit DNA from their parents that leaves them at risk of cancer.

With its focus centered so squarely on all aspects of DNA, genomic care is ideally positioned to tackle both acquired and inherited genes that go awry, giving doctors a powerful new set of anti-cancer weapons. Healthy people who wonder if certain types of cancer run in their family can now take genetic tests that assess their own personal level of risk, letting them take preventive steps if that risk is high.

People already diagnosed with cancer, like Parker, can increasingly have their tumors profiled, revealing genes that spell out a tumor's identity, features—and weaknesses. Many doctors say the information in these profiles represents the genomic equivalent of unmasking a killer, making it far easier to understand a tumor and fight it. In some cases, these cancer profiles even point the way to innovative, targeted medicines that can shrink or kill tumors with fewer side effects than traditional radiation or chemotherapy.

If you are worried about developing cancer, or have cancer, genomic medicine doesn't yet hold all the answers. But genomic advances against cancer are moving quickly. Cancer comes in hundreds of forms—more than we can cover in detail here. But as genomic tools become the future of finding, treating, and even preventing cancer, you'll find a growing body of answers to your own cancer questions. If multiple types of cancer have occurred in your family, for example, a genetic counselor armed with new insights may be able to help you uncover important underlying genetic patterns and help you protect your family's health.

This chapter looks at some of the biggest ways genomic medicine is strengthening your hand against cancer. We cover some of the innovations in tests and treatments, and also look at where these tools fit in the options for addressing some of the more common malignancies. To get started, let's go back to your DNA, and look at its potential for morphing into an agent of cancer.

DNA AND CANCER

What we commonly call cancer is actually at least 200 different diseases. While these illnesses affect many different parts of the body, they all arise from the same starting point—DNA changes that alter the normal growth, division, and death of cells.

Here's how these errant genes get their start. As you may recall from Chapter 1, your DNA carries the instructions for how your body functions, builds itself, and repairs itself. Some of your DNA carries the code that spells out how your cells—your body's basic work units—divide and copy themselves. These copies are necessary for you to grow new cells, replace old ones, or repair damaged tissue. When it comes time for your cells to make these new copies of themselves, they usually operate under gene instructions that guide the process in a controlled, predictable way. If you burn your arm, for example, specific genes in your body order certain cells to copy themselves rapidly until new tissue is formed, the damage is repaired, and the burn is healed. Once the injury is past, those same cells return to their normal rate of division.

But sometimes, the DNA that controls cell division and growth gets damaged. This dangerous mutation then becomes part of the cell's code, often triggering a cascading series of gene mistakes that outstrip your genome's abilities to repair itself. As further cells are copied from the damaged one, they will all contain that same mutation.

Some of these altered cells, while busy dividing abnormally, never become more than minor menaces. They simply stay put in their original tissue. They may grow abnormally, piling up in a lumpy unstructured mass that looks odd or presses on other parts of the body. But these growths, called benign tumors, often don't cause any broader health problems. While benign tumors can sometimes grow quite large, they are often relatively easy to remove and treat. Sometimes, doctors even opt to leave them in place.

Other tumors don't sit harmlessly in one spot. If cells acquire a sufficient number of mutations, they begin acting even more abnormally, gaining the ability not only to grow, but also to spread. These aggressive growths are true cancers. Called malignant tumors, these cancers not only destroy the tissue where they first arose, but invade other parts of the body. A look at the unique features that tumors must gain to become malignant shows just how complex cancer is—and all the gene-driven mechanisms doctors have to tackle in controlling it:

Cancer Gets Its Own Genome Project

Now that a healthy human genome has been spelled out, scientists are turning their attention to damaged forms of DNA. In an offshoot of the Human Genome Project, scientists with the National Cancer Institute have created a research project called the Cancer Genome Atlas. This project is working to create a map of all the gene changes involved with cancer; the ultimate goal is for better cancer prevention, diagnosis, and treatment. The project started by analyzing three relatively common malignancies—lung, brain, and ovarian cancer. In a few years, you'll probably see improved weapons against these cancers thanks to this project.

- While most normal cells need signals from outside the cell before they start growing, cells that are becoming cancerous don't need to wait. They are able to generate many of their own growth signals.
- Cells that are becoming cancerous also become insensitive to signals that typically tell a cell to stop growing.
- Most normal cells have a system of programmed death. But cells that are becoming cancerous can skirt this self-destruct mechanism.
- Most normal cells carry built-in limits on their ability to multiply. Cells that are becoming cancerous, however, can ignore those restrictions, as well.
- As they grow and multiply abnormally, cells on their way to becoming cancerous develop the ability to encourage new blood vessel growth to keep themselves nourished.
- These steps add up to the ultimate hallmark of malignant tumors— the ability to move through the body and grow in new tissues.

Once these growths invade new tissue, they usually repeat their destructive habits, destroying other cells and growing out of control. These growths are called metastatic tumors. As cancer spreads, or metastasizes, in this way, doctors often find they have fewer options for stopping it.

Because it arises from damaged DNA, cancer is always considered a gene-driven disease. All cases of cancer arise from acquired mutations— probably somewhere between four to seven mutations in key genes that affect important parts of your cell's growth cycle. But it's important to note that though cancer happens as a result of DNA changes, these mutations are not usually inherited. Only about 10 percent of people have a single inherited predisposition that significantly increases their risk of cancer. Other people may not have genetic variants linked to cancer so clearly, but they may carry less powerful variants that increase their risk when certain external factors, such as toxins in cigarette smoke, are present.

Our lives, unfortunately, contain plenty of these risk factors. Unhealthy diets high in fat and low in fresh fruits and vegetables, along with daily routines short on exercise, play a role in the DNA damage that gives rise to cancer. Some infectious diseases trigger mutations, such as the human papillomavirus (HPV) that can give rise to cervical cancer. Excess exposure to ultraviolet light from the sun or sunlamps can harm the DNA in your skin. Hazardous chemicals such as asbestos or benzene, a cancer-causing agent used in industrial workplaces and found in cigarette smoke, can also disrupt human DNA. Common tobacco products, such as cigarettes and cigars, pack so many cancerous chemicals that genomic scientists increasingly consider them a leading source of DNA damage. Scientists estimate that about 30 percent of the 1.4 million cancers discovered in Americans each year could be eliminated by lifestyle changes.

Cancer is a serious illness, and preventing it should be a top health priority for each of us. But amid all the fear surrounding cancer, there are also hopeful signs that are worth noting. Overall, deaths from cancer are

Common Sense Health Advice: It's Good for Your Genes, Too

We've all heard the standard suggestions for good health many times—don't smoke, eat right, and exercise. But did you know these truisms go deeper than general well being? They can actually help keep your DNA healthy and prevent the genomic damage that leads to cancer. Here's how:

- By avoiding tobacco, you dodge the cancer-causing chemicals in cigarettes that have been linked to tumors of the lungs, throat, bladder, and many other parts of the body. If you smoke, these DNA destroyers not only fill your body, but also waft into the lungs of your family and others who breathe in your second-hand smoke. Kicking the habit can be tough, but your genes—and the genes of your family and friends—will thank you.
- By eating a balanced diet rich in brightly colored fruits and vegetables, you help your genes fend off harmful intruders. Antioxidants, healthful substances that appear to mop up DNA-damaging particles in the body, are found in abundance in these foods. Think twice, though, before you try to boost your antioxidant levels higher by taking lots of vitamin supplements. In some studies, people who took high levels of supplemental antioxidants encountered unexpected health problems.
- By getting at least 30 minutes of exercise a day, you help your body and your genes stay in balance. By increasing your metabolism, regulating your hormones, and keeping you trimmer, exercise has proven to reduce a person's risk of a wide variety of common cancers. In one study of breast cancer risk alone, women at normal risk for breast cancer who got at least four hours of exercise a week during their reproductive years had more than a 50 percent reduction in their cancer risk.
- It may be fashionable to tan, but your skin pays a heavy price. Ultraviolet rays damage skin cells and their DNA. And with serious burns or continuous exposure, that DNA has a hard time repairing itself. Exposure before age 18, when the body is still developing, can be most harmful, but sun exposure at any age can increase your risk of developing skin cancer. Minimizing sun exposure and using sunscreen decrease your risk substantially.

In being healthful, these simple guidelines turn out to be good for the whole of you, right down to helping to keep your DNA free of cancer-causing mistakes.

now dropping. While plenty of people are still being diagnosed with cancer, more of them are surviving, often with the help of genomic innovation. Many of these improvements may go unnoticed in our everyday routines; one advance may boost hope in a particular type of cancer here, while another may save a few lives there. In the fight against cervical cancer, for example, a relatively recent genetic test that detects a cancer-related virus is quickly becoming the best way to catch cervical cancer early. Bit by bit, such innovations are adding up to a revolution in preventing and treating this serious disease.

Cutting Cancer's Power to Kill

Cancer remains a scary disease, but improved detection and treatment—including advances in genomic medicine—are helping more and more people survive it:

- Of the 1.4 million new cases each year, about 1 million are skin cancers that are now highly curable.
- Overall, the five-year survival rate for all cancers is about 65 percent—up 15 percent from 20 years ago.
- The five-year survival rate for breast cancers that haven't migrated beyond breast tissue is now 98 percent.
- The five-year survival rate for prostate cancer at any stage of severity is now close to 100 percent.

Genomic scientists are working to help people with other types of cancer share in these more optimistic numbers. Ultimately, by improving our understanding of how this disease develops, they hope far fewer people will ever have to worry about dying from cancer.

First we take a broader look at some of the major genomic innovations in cancer, and then discuss how these advances affect a few specific forms of the condition.

Genetic Testing for Cancer Risk

While cancer is always triggered by acquired mutations, inherited genetic factors can also play a role in increasing your risk. Some inherited gene mutations are rare, but also increase risk to a greater degree. Other inherited genetic factors are more common, but do less to boost risk. Cancer risk testing is available for both types of genetic factors.

Testing for the first type of risk factors is best suited to people from families or ethnic groups known to carry these risk factors. Some families, for example, carry mutations that greatly increase their risk of developing cancer, including particular types of breast, ovarian, colorectal, skin, and pancreatic malignancies. While most people don't carry these mutations, about 5 to 10 percent of individuals with these cancers have their disease as a result of an inherited predisposition mutation. The best-known of these genetic factors are *BRCA1* and *BRCA2*, which are discussed in more detail later in this chapter. Certain mutations in the *BRCA* genes have been linked to greatly increased risk of breast and ovarian cancer.

More recently, newer forms of genetic testing also look for more common, less powerful genetic variants linked to cancer risk. These tests provide less definitive answers about risk, but they cover more forms of cancer, including prostate cancer, lung cancer, and more common types of breast cancer and colorectal cancer. If you undergo this type of testing for breast cancer risk, for example, your analysis will probably cover several locations on your genome known to have some link to breast cancer, but it won't analyze your *BRCA* genes.

Common Types of Cancer in the United States

Men	Genetic Link or Test
Bladder	Certain genetic factors known to increase risk in some cases; targeted drugs in development
Colon and rectum	Genetic risk tests available; targeted drugs in use and in development
Kidney	Genetic factors can increase risk; targeted drugs available and in development
Leukemia	Genetic factors can increase risk; profiling tests available or in development
Lung and bronchus	Genetic risk is relatively low; targeted drugs in use and in development
Melanoma	Genetic risk test available in some cases; one significant gene therapy breakthrough
Mouth and throat	Genetic factors can increase risk; new diagnostic saliva test for oral cancer in development
Non-Hodgkin lymphoma	DNA profiling tests available; targeted drugs available and in development
Pancreas	Genetic risk test available in some cases; targeted drugs in development
Prostate	SNP-based risk testing is available, but isn't definitive

Women	Genetic Link or Test
Breast	Genetic risk test available; profiling tests available; targeted drugs available
Bladder	Certain genes known to increase risk in some cases; targeted drugs in development
Colon and rectum	Genetic risk tests available; targeted drugs in use and in development
Lung and bronchus	Genetic risk is relatively low; targeted drugs in use and in development
Melanoma	Genetic risk test available in some cases; one significant gene therapy breakthrough
Non-Hodgkin lymphoma	DNA profiling available; targeted drugs available and in development
Ovary	Genetic risk test available; targeted drugs in development
Pancreas	Genetic risk test available in some cases; targeted drugs in development
Thyroid	Genetic risk is low; targeted drugs in development
Uterine corpus	HNPCC, a colon cancer risk mutation, can also boost risk for this cancer

When Risk Testing Can Help

Genetic testing for cancer risk is most informative for those who come from a family with a lot of cancer or a background linked to higher rates of certain types of cancer. These tests are now available for mutations linked to some cases of breast cancer, colorectal cancer, ovarian cancer, pancreatic cancer, and melanoma, an aggressive form of skin cancer. Doctors usually reserve these tests for people known to have a higher risk, who sometimes turn to them to test before any signs of the disease arise, in the hopes of preventing cancer before it starts or detecting the cancer at the earliest stage possible.

Typically, this type of genetic risk test begins by evaluating your family history (see Chapter 2). Using information about the types of cancer and the ages at which they arose in your family, your doctor or genetic counselor can perform a risk assessment to identify which genes are more likely to be involved in increasing the cancer risk in your family. For example, of the two most common genetic variants that predispose a person to certain inherited forms of colon cancer, the type of cancers, the ages at which they occur, and even the pathology of the colon cancers are different in families, depending on which gene variant is inherited. In addition, your doctor or genetic counselor can also identify who is the

How Do I Tell My Family?

Few topics can be more important—or more difficult—than sharing concerns about inherited cancer risk with your family. If you've had a positive test for inherited cancer risk, this information is vital for your relatives' health. But it may be difficult to discuss. While many families band together during risk testing, the idea of cancer is still frightening, and conversations about shared risk can be confusing and stressful. And in families that aren't close, telling estranged relatives that they may have an increased risk of developing cancer can be extremely difficult.

Still, these conversations are worth the effort. Your family's health may depend on them. Here are some considerations that can make these discussions go a little more smoothly:

- Your family may share genes, but not the same views on examining them. Your decision to get tested was right for you. But some members of your family may not be emotionally ready to undergo a test themselves. This can be frustrating, but it's their choice, just as your test was your decision.
- Don't be surprised if your news steers the conversation in unexpected directions. Relatives who hear of your test results may come forth with medical information they were reluctant or embarrassed to share before. While these revelations can be surprising or even upsetting, they can also contribute important information to your family medical history.
- Think carefully about how and when to tell your children. Your test affects them as well, and can start shaping their own health care early in life. Remember, young children often don't understand complicated genomic concepts, and teenagers may not always be emotionally ready to cope with the news, especially if a parent has cancer. Typically, testing children isn't advised unless there is something specific that will change in the child's health care—for example, in one type of colon cancer, it is recommended that children with a deleterious mutation have their first colonoscopy before age 15. Talk with your genetic counselor, who often has experience in helping families inform children of inherited medical risks or conditions. Some genomic health centers also offer support groups for children and teenagers with genetic risks or illness in their family.
- Make sure you communicate your news clearly. While most people prefer to have conversations about family genetics in person or over the phone, these conversations are usually emotional. It can be hard to make sure each person you tell receives and remembers all the medical information they need. It's often a good idea to follow up conversations with a simple letter that outlines your test results, explains what they may mean, and summarizes what steps your relatives can take to assess their own risks. Many genetic counselors help their patients draft these letters. If you'd like to see examples of similar letters written in relation to breast cancer risk, visit www.myriadtests.com/results.htm, where a leading genetic testing company offers sample letters for patients to consider.

No matter how tricky these conversations seem, remember that you don't have to address them unprepared. Talk to your genetic counselor, who has experience in helping families share even the most difficult genetic news.

most appropriate testing candidate in your family. The person most likely to reveal any inherited genetic factors is typically someone who has developed cancer already. Once an inherited mutation has been identified in one family member, your doctor or genetic counselor can help identify other at-risk family members.

If you are thinking about a genetic test for cancer risk, the National Cancer Institute recommends considering the following questions first, both on your own and with your doctor or genetic counselor:

- What are the chances that an inherited gene alteration is involved in any cancer in my family or me?
- If there is an inherited gene alteration in my family, what are my chances that I have it?
- What are my reasons for wanting to be tested?
- Besides having altered genes, what are my other risk factors for developing cancer?
- How much does the test cost? How long will it take to get my results?
- What are the possible results of the test?
- What would a positive result mean for me?
- What would a negative result mean for me?
- Do I want to ask my insurance company to pay for my test?
- Where will my test results be placed/recorded? Who will have access to them?
- Would knowing this information cause my family members or me to make changes in medical care?
- What type of cancer screening is recommended if I don't get tested?

In addition to helping you decide on testing, your answers to these questions can also help you make plans for handling your test results, should you decide to go ahead with the analysis.

If you don't come from a family or background with a link to these types of mutations, you may still choose to undergo SNP-based cancer risk testing. This form of testing is most commonly offered by commercial genetic testing companies that either work through doctors or sell their tests directly to the public. These tests focus on different DNA, usually looking at SNPs that are more common but have a less powerful effect on cancer risk.

The Limits of Risk Testing

The limits of cancer risk testing reflect which type of testing you undergo—analysis for more rare mutations with a stronger effect, or analysis for SNPs that are more common but have a smaller effect on risk.

If you undergo the first type of testing for a mutation in a gene such as *BRCA1* or *BRCA2*, here are several limitations to keep in mind:

- Having a mutation increases your risk of developing cancer. But it's important to remember that, while this higher risk should be taken seriously, it's no guarantee that you'll develop a malignancy.
- If you are a member of a family with a known inherited mutation and your test shows you aren't at increased risk, that can be great news. It's important to remember, though, that a negative test doesn't mean you face no risk of cancer. Your risks remain at least the same as those of the general population. Even if your test is negative, you'll still need to follow general guidelines on cancer prevention and screening.

Failing to Share Genetic Information Can Hurt Others

"How could they do this to me? What did I ever do to them that would make them hate me this much?" As Katie cried in my office, my heart fell to my stomach. Recognizing her specific mutation, I realized that I had been the genetic counselor for her family members three years ago. I knew the family was estranged, but could I have prevented Katie's cancer by pushing the family harder to share their genetic information?

Katie had been diagnosed with colon cancer at age 39, and because she was young, she was offered genetic testing. Today was the result session, and she was prepared to learn that she had an inherited mutation. It would partly explain why she developed cancer at such a young age. For many people with cancer, learning that they have a mutation can be reassuring because it seems to lessen their sense of having done something to cause the cancer. It was her family's betrayal that she found painful, because her colon cancer might have been prevented if they had shared their test results with her three years ago.

Katie's dad was the black sheep of the family. A family feud that he never discussed had resulted in estrangement. She had met the family only once, about 15 years ago. She knew they lived locally, but his sisters were married and had different last names.

During the initial genetic consultation, Katie had provided lots of information about her mother's side of the family. But her father had died in an accident 10 years before, and she really didn't know anything about his family. Between the time she had blood drawn and learned her result, Katie's mom had done some searching and discovered that her estranged husband's sisters and their father had also had cancer. One sister had colon cancer at age 49, the other had endometrial cancer, and their father died of colon cancer in his late fifties. This was a classic Lynch syndrome family.

Katie's aunts had been tested and learned of their mutation about three years ago. But their brother, who they never liked, was dead, and although they were encouraged to tell their sister-in-law (I reviewed my letter and had included that piece, thankfully!) they hadn't communicated with her. Katie's siblings scheduled colonoscopies after learning of her diagnosis, and her older brother had four polyps removed. However, her aunts' decision to withhold information had hurt Katie—both physically and emotionally.

Bottom line: As a genetic counselor, I encourage patients to communicate information about genetic status with families, especially when there is a mutation that could affect someone's decisions about medical care. Often during counseling sessions, we learn of family estrangements and help create model letters or explore other ways to share the information with extended family members at risk. Once the health care provider clarifies who should be told, it is the family's responsibility to share the information. Even if you don't like your brother, his kids don't deserve to develop a cancer that may have been avoided with proactive medical care.

- If you do get tested, you'll have to contend with the fact that this type of cancer risk testing can't always provide definitive answers. Even in families with an identifiable mutation, testing usually provides information only about the chances of developing cancer—not predictions on if or exactly when the disease will arise. Most often, cancer-linked mutations only point to an increased risk of the disease. To be sure, this increased risk can be quite high—certain mutations linked to breast cancer, for example, give a woman a 60 to 80 percent chance that she'll develop this type of cancer by the time she is 70. But those risk numbers are for a 70-year-old woman who hasn't done anything to reduce her risk. If you learn whether you carry a cancer-linked mutation, you can consider preventive measures to lower that risk.
- Remember that these tests aren't designed to examine the risks for people in the general population. They detect only certain mutations most commonly found in particular families in which there are many individuals with cancer or in individuals with specific types of cancers. Some ethnic groups, such as people with Eastern European Ashkenazi Jewish ancestry, have an increased chance of having particular mutations that can be easily analyzed. For this reason, doctors usually recommend genetic cancer risk testing only to people with these characteristic cancers, from families with significant histories of cancer, or particular ethnic backgrounds. If you aren't sure if you represent a good match for a cancer risk test, talk to your doctor or make an appointment with a genetic counselor who specializes in assessing familial cancer risk. They can help you determine if you are a good fit for this type of cancer risk testing.
- There's also a small chance that your test could miss your mutation. The possibility of receiving a false negative test result is small. But our understanding of cancer-linked genes is still developing, and that means test results may not always tell the correct story. Some families, for example, may have a mutation that boosts their risk but doesn't precisely match other cancer-linked mutations that have already been clearly identified. In other families, analysis of the wrong gene may have occurred. If your test results seem at odds with your family or medical history, talk to your genetic counselor. You may want to review your family history in more detail, or talk about your options for additional testing.

If you undergo the second type of testing for cancer-related SNPs, there are several limitations worth considering, as well:

- The SNPs analyzed in this form of testing have a smaller effect on cancer risk. Knowing your SNP-based risk won't tell you definitely whether or not you'll develop cancer.
- Your test will not cover every possible cancer-related SNP in your genome. The SNPs analyzed by these tests vary from company to

company. And scientists are still working to discover all the SNPs related to cancer risk in the human genome.

- A low risk score on one of these tests is no guarantee of a cancer-free future. Your test may not have looked at SNPs that aren't yet recognized as important. These tests also don't cover genetic variations with a stronger effect, such as *BRCA*. And many cancers still occur as a result of environmental damage that may have little to do with your inherited genetic risk. You'll still need to be mindful of preventing and watching for cancer.

If you aren't sure about any of the cancer risk tests currently available, remember that these tests aren't your only option. A detailed family medical history can often reveal whether a pattern of cancer runs in your bloodline, and could turn out to be reassuring if it reveals that your risk may be lower than you thought. You can also talk to your doctor about how your age, your diet, your work, and your lifestyle affect your cancer risk. By undergoing regular cancer screenings and following basic cancer-prevention guidelines, you can reduce your risks of cancer without ever taking a genetic test.

Special Considerations for Risk Testing

Some people considering cancer risk testing are understandably nervous. Test results that show high risk can be frightening. But this information, while daunting, also offers hope. Some people learn that they do not have the mutation seen in other family members and receive peace of mind in knowing that their risk is essentially the same as that of the general population. For those with a mutation or risk-related SNP, knowing your risk lets you start a preventive program to ward off cancer or help catch it early, when it is far easier to treat. In some cases, these measures are relatively simple, such as getting screening tests more frequently or starting them at an earlier age. In others, preventive measures are more drastic. Some people who have an increased risk of cancer choose preventive surgery to remove the organs at risk for developing the disease, such as their colons, breasts, or ovaries. While such an operation might seem extreme, those who choose this option say they prefer surgery to the prospect of cancer later in life. For families with a strong history of cancer, these tests and preventive steps often offer relief after generations of worry.

If you choose any form of cancer risk testing, be sure to pursue your test through a service that provides genetic counseling. Cancer risk information is complex, and some people find it confusing or even overwhelming. By seeking a genetic counselor's help in interpreting your results, you'll have a much clearer picture of your risk and be able to make more informed decisions about protecting your health.

In the past, some people considering cancer risk testing were especially concerned about the issue of genetic discrimination. If their test

Cautions in Cancer Risk Testing

When it comes to direct-to-consumer testing for genetic cancer risks, gene experts have simple advice: Get help. These tests are complicated, with powerful implications for your health.

If you find that you are curious about a direct-to-consumer cancer risk test, here are three questions that can help you make a more informed choice:

- What does this test analyze? Not all cancer risk tests are created equally. Is the science behind the test credible? How many genetic factors does the test assess? Don't waste your time or money on a test that doesn't look for anything proven or useful, or where the value of the test isn't clear to you.
- How much will it cost? Tests for cancer risk are expensive, often starting in the hundreds of dollars. Tests for mutations in genes such as *BRCA1* and *BRCA2* usually cost more than $2,000. Find out if your insurance plan will help cover the costs of testing.
- How will you know what the results mean? Cancer risk tests aren't easy to understand—sometimes even for genetic experts. If you choose a direct-to-consumer test, select one that comes with the services of a board-certified genetic counselor.

If you do choose a direct-to-consumer test, plan on sharing your results with your doctor, no matter what. Information on your cancer risk will be the most valuable if experts help you understand how to use it to protect your health.

results showed high risk, they feared, that information could not only wind up in their own medical records but also in those of their families. Recent federal legal protections, however, prevent many forms of genetic discrimination. You'll find more information on this topic in Chapter 8.

The Bottom Line on Risk Testing

Genetic cancer risk testing may be a good choice if certain forms of inherited cancer run in your family, if you come from a particular ethnic background, or if you'd like some sense of your SNP-based risk. But talk to your doctor and a genetic counselor before taking such a test, and seek their expertise in understanding and acting on your results. If you do opt for a direct-to-consumer genetic testing company, select one that offers the support of licensed genetic counselors. Your results will be more understandable and useful if you have a counselor's help.

UNDERSTANDING YOUR CANCER'S PROFILE

If you've already received a diagnosis of cancer, your doctor may be able to offer you a new opportunity to scrutinize the genes driving your illness—information that may make those rogue stretches of DNA easier to stop. In a growing number of cancer cases, including breast cancer and lymphoma, doctors can now use genomic technology to create a detailed molecular portrait of an individual cancer. This technology goes far beyond traditional methods of analyzing tumors, which classify cancer by the general appearance of a tumor and its surrounding tissue. These new tools analyze a cancer's DNA, providing information on thousands of cancer genes and their activity patterns all at once. By creating this cancer profile, doctors can increasingly determine the potential for the cancer to spread, the chances of the cancer recurring, and what medicines might best stop the malignancy.

When Cancer Profiling Can Help

Cancer profiling has made it clear that cancers we typically lump together by location—breast cancer or lymph cancer for example—actually come in many distinct forms. These different varieties have their own identities, habits, and weaknesses, and knowing their details can sometimes give you a big boost in your fight against cancer. Tumor profiles are now used in the treatment of many different types of cancer. In addition to the form of breast cancer recurrence profiling described at the start of this chapter, for example, blood cancer specialists are increasingly turning to profiles to better understand sub-types of lymphoma.

The Limits of Cancer Profiling

Cancer profiling is still an emerging field of cancer care, limiting its availability. If you have cancer, you may find that molecular profiles aren't yet widely available for the type of cancer you have. Or you may find that profiles for your type of cancer are only available by enrolling in research studies, and the timing of the research study may not match your own treatment needs. Sometimes, your doctors may not yet be comfortable entrusting your care to tools that are this new. Not all cancer specialists agree that cancer profiles are ready for widespread use, and some prefer to rely on traditional analysis and treatments rather than take risks with newer options.

If you are able to have your cancer profiled, you'll also likely find that these profiles don't always offer clear yes or no answers on which course of treatment to follow. Instead, cancer profiles more often talk about risk and likelihood. Parker Lee, for example, learned that her cancer had a very low likelihood of returning—less than 10 percent. That figure is small, but it's not the same as having a risk report of zero. Parker and her doctor decided they were comfortable making a treatment decision in the face of some risk. But not everyone would be. If you are considering cancer profiling, both you and your doctor need to consider the level of uncertainty you are willing to accept.

If you do undergo profiling, you may also have to face the fact that cancer profiles don't always offer the news you'd like to hear. Your profile could show that your cancer is easily treated or unlikely to return, or point out which drugs might best control it. But your tumor's profile could also reveal an aggressive cancer that won't respond well to current treatments. This disappointing news can be hard to take amid all the emotional ups and downs that come with a cancer diagnosis. Keep in mind, though, that even a discouraging profile can offer useful insights. If your cancer won't respond well to regular treatment, for example, your tumor profile may make you a good candidate for experimental therapies.

Before your cancer is profiled, think carefully about how you'll handle any bad news. Talk to your doctors, family, and caregivers ahead of time, so they can support you once you learn your cancer's profile.

Special Considerations for Cancer Profiling

This area of genomic medicine offers no do-it-yourself options. If you are considering cancer profiling, you'll need the support of your doctor to obtain this kind of cancer analysis and act on its results. Not all cancer specialists are comfortable with the idea of making medical decisions based on the results of molecular cancer profiles. So it's important that you and your doctor share similar views on cancer profiling.

If you are interested in cancer profiling, talk to your cancer caregivers about their own experience with the procedure. Are they familiar with what profiles are available for your type of cancer? Have they used them before? Is your type of cancer one for which genetic profiling would provide additional information? If so, are they willing to help you make medical decisions based on your profile results? Or do they consider this technology too new to be reliable or useful?

Sometimes, even with all the interest in profiles among cancer specialists, you may find that your doctors don't consider a tumor profile to be one of your best options. This is especially true when it comes to using a tumor profile to make treatment decisions for some types of cancer. Some doctors, for example, would have strongly disagreed with Parker Lee's decision to skip chemotherapy, arguing that when it comes to breast cancer, it's best to play it safe. If you aren't sure about your doctors' views on tumor profiles, you can certainly seek other medical opinions. But it's worth giving different points of view careful consideration. If you plan to make treatment decisions based on your cancer profile, it's

Finding a Cancer Clinical Trial

If you've been diagnosed with cancer and want to find out about emerging gene-based tests or treatments, the best place to start is with the National Cancer Institute's list of ongoing cancer clinical trials. You can find an up-to-date list online, at www.cancer.gov/clinicaltrials. That section of the NCI's Web site also offers a detailed guide to finding and enrolling in many different types of clinical trials. Among the guide's key pointers:

- If you are newly diagnosed with cancer and interested in a clinical trial, talk to your doctors immediately. Many trials only take patients during a specific time in treatment—sometimes even before any treatment starts. Learning which trials are available at various times during your treatment can ensure that you don't delay regular care if waiting could harm you, and might possibly still give you clinical trial options at a later time.
- If you find an appropriate trial that sounds promising, make sure you get a copy of a document called the protocol summary. This is the trial's action plan, and will help you and your doctor decide if the trial is a good fit for you.
- Filling out clinical trial applications or enrollment forms can be complicated. Ask a nurse or patient advocate at your doctor's office for help. Sometimes, the study coordinators for the trial can also help with the enrollment forms.

Most people don't learn about clinical trials until they need special treatment. But it's best to become informed about trials earlier, so that you can make quick, educated decisions should you or your family ever consider specialized care. Take some time to learn about the general concepts of clinical trials before a diagnosis even happens. You'll find more information on clinical trials in Chapter 9 and the Resources section of this book.

important to weigh many opinions, from the traditional to the cutting-edge, beforehand.

The Bottom Line on Cancer Profiling

Cancer profiles increasingly offer a way for you and your doctors to create a detailed portrait of your cancer, revealing its patterns and weaknesses. They aren't yet available for all types of cancer, but if they are an option for your cancer care, they can offer you vital information. Talk to your doctors about profiling and what benefits a tumor analysis may hold for you. You can also review the National Cancer Institute's ongoing list of clinical trials in cancer to see if any scientists are offering new or experimental profiles for your type of cancer. You'll find more information on this list of trials in the Resources section at the back of this book.

TARGETING YOUR TREATMENTS FOR CANCER

New abilities to profile cancer sometimes bring new choices for treating it. These new medicines target particular features of certain

Cancer Yields to a Gene Therapy Breakthrough

Gene therapy—healing gene-based diseases by repairing damaged DNA—remains a key goal of genomic medicine. So far, it's proven very difficult to tinker with human genes safely or effectively. But in studies of melanoma, a very serious type of skin cancer, scientists have won an important victory in their push for gene therapy. They rebuilt important immune cells in a handful of patients with this aggressive form of skin cancer, with some hopeful results.

The breakthrough came in a small study of 17 melanoma patients. Scientists took disease-fighting white blood cells from these patients, and rebuilt the cells using proteins that help them find, attack, and destroy cancer cells. To their delight, two of the 17 patients saw their cancer virtually disappear. And none of the patients suffered serious side effects from their rebuilt cells—a major concern in gene therapy.

Big questions remain after this experiment. Why didn't the other 15 patients also improve? Why, in these patients, did many of the rebuilt white blood cells disappear within a month? Can this type of immune boost work against other cancers?

This research and the larger issue of gene therapy are discussed in more detail in Chapter 9. After years of starts and stops in gene therapy, this small victory in the fight against cancer may have cracked open the door to one of the most hopeful goals of genomic medicine.

cancers, often choking off their ability to grow or blocking their spread through the body. Such targeted therapies are being developed quickly for many common types of cancer, including lung cancer, blood cancers, and breast cancer.

Each of these treatments starts with tests that measure either certain gene-driven features of a tumor or a small piece of a person's DNA that affects their response to a particular medication. Herceptin, a targeted medication for breast cancer, is one such drug. When used against the types of tumors Herceptin is designed to treat, the drug blocks the output of a particular gene that drives tumor growth. Herceptin also makes it easier for your body's immune system to destroy cancer cells. If you have breast cancer, your doctor can tell if Herceptin is right for you by testing the activity of just one of your cancer's genes.

Another promising targeted drug is Avastin, a medication first approved to fight colorectal cancer. Avastin works by targeting a protein called VEGF, which stimulates the formation of new blood vessels—including the blood vessels cancer cells need to grow and spread. Limiting the growth of these blood vessels shuts down a tumor's ability to multiply, slowly starving it of vital oxygen and nutrients. Avastin is now being used against many other types of tumors. Some of those specific uses are covered later in this chapter.

When Targeted Treatment Can Help

If available for your type of cancer, targeted therapies may offer major improvements in slowing or reversing your illness. Some of these treatments also make it far less likely that your cancer will return. While these new medications haven't helped every cancer patient who has tried them, their gains have been impressive enough to persuade doctors to adopt them quickly. Some targeted therapies approved for use against one type of cancer, such as Herceptin, are now being considered for use against other cancers, boosting the chances that there will be some sort of targeted therapy available for you to try.

In addition to the boost they bring in fighting cancer, these treatments are also often easier on your body. While they may still have side effects, targeted treatments may be less grueling than other therapies long used against cancer, such as chemotherapy or radiation.

The Limits of Targeted Treatment

Targeted therapies aren't yet available for every type of cancer. They often work only on sub-types of a particular cancer—certain types of breast tumors or lung cancers, for example. They're also more likely to be used against aggressive cancers. If your cancer doesn't match the profile of any targeted medications, you'll have to fall back on more conventional treatments. While traditional cancer medicines and therapies have strong track records of their own, some people may be disappointed when they find their cancer doesn't fit the profile for targeted therapy.

It's also important to remember that targeted therapies aren't a magic bullet. Many have shown impressive abilities to fight cancer. But they don't work in every patient who tries them. Cancer is a very complicated set of diseases, and even the most innovative medicines can't offer any guarantees.

Targeted medicines also don't eliminate the need for standard treatments such as surgery, chemotherapy, or radiation. Almost all breast cancer patients who use Herceptin, for example, also undergo tumor-removal surgery or mastectomy. Herceptin is also usually used in combination with chemotherapy. Your doctor will want to use every available tool to fight your cancer, making it unlikely that targeted drugs will let you bypass standard cancer treatments.

Special Considerations of Targeted Treatment

Some targeted cancer treatments are very expensive, often costing tens of thousands of dollars for a full course of tests and drugs. However, if your cancer matches the profile for one of these medications, your medical insurance will usually cover some or all of the cost. Talk to your doctor or insurer beforehand, so that you know whether a targeted drug will mean money out of your own pocket.

While these treatments are usually reserved for patients who match the drug's profile, some others ask their doctor to try the medication anyway, hoping for any boost in their cancer fight. A few doctors, sympathetic to this desire to try every possible option, have agreed to use targeted drugs in such cases. Most doctors, however, won't, citing the fact that they are not proven, the high cost, and the toll any cancer treatment takes on a person's body. It's also important to keep in mind that insurance companies usually won't cover such uses of targeted treatments. If you'd like to try a targeted cancer therapy, but don't fit the drug's profile, you'll probably have to cover the costs yourself.

The Bottom Line on Targeted Treatments

Targeted medicines are a great ally in fighting some types of cancer, and as new tumor profiles are developed, more targeted treatments will be developed to match them. But these treatments are not yet available for all types of cancer. Remember that if your cancer doesn't fit a drug's profile, you can still fall back on more conventional treatments. Targeted therapies can be a big boost, but they aren't your only source of hope.

GENOMICS AND BREAST CANCER

Breast cancer strikes more than 200,000 women in the United States each year, making it the second most common form of cancer among women. More than 40,000 women die from breast cancer each year, and men can be diagnosed with it as well. Cancer can arise anywhere in breast tissue, but the most dangerous tumors are those that spread beyond breast tissue and metastasize in other parts of the body.

The causes of breast cancer are still unknown. A woman's hormones, medications, diet, and lifestyle all appear to play a role. But in about 5 to 10 percent of all breast cancer cases, genetic inheritance also has a clear effect, led by particular genetic mutations that greatly increase breast cancer risk. In other cases, more common but less powerful genetic variants also appear to increase risk, although to a smaller degree.

Because breast cancer is common, it has been the focus of intense genomic research. As a result, more genomic advances have been made in breast cancer than any other type of malignancy. Women concerned about breast cancer risk, or who have developed the disease, have various options for risk screening, tumor profiling, and targeted treatment.

Genetic Testing for Breast Cancer Risk

The role of inherited genetic factors can vary widely. In many cases of the condition, inherited factors appear to

---

Did You Know ?

*B*RCA mutations aren't the only genetic variations linked to breast cancer. Other genes, called *CHEK2*, *ATM*, and *BRIP1*, can also increase a woman's risk of breast cancer, although far less than *BRCA1* or *BRCA2* mutations. Like *BRCA* mutations, these genetic factors are involved in DNA repair—a good indication that impaired abilities to fix gene damage are an important factor in breast cancer. It's likely that scientists will continue to uncover more breast cancer mutations, making more genetic tests for breast cancer risk likely in the years ahead.

contribute to risk, but do not emerge as the dominant cause. In these more common forms of the condition, scientists estimate that about 30 percent of risk is genetic.

In about 5 to 10 percent of all breast cancer cases, however, that risk estimate jumps substantially. These cases are most commonly linked to increased cancer susceptibility genes called *BRCA1*, located on Chromosome 17, and *BRCA2*, located on Chromosome 13. These genes, considered tumor suppressor genes, typically stop cells from growing out of control. Mutations in these genes make it easier for normal genes to develop into cancerous ones. Women with these *BRCA* mutations have a 60 to 80 percent chance of developing breast cancer by age 70.

If you want to learn whether you carry a *BRCA* mutation, the best place to start is your family medical history. Most women with *BRCA* mutations have what gene experts call a significant family history of breast cancer. This is defined as having two or more close family members (a mother, daughter, sister, grandmother, or aunt) with breast cancer, at least one of which was diagnosed before age 50. However, since gene mutations can also be inherited from your father's side of the family, it is important to evaluate that side, as well.

When *BRCA* mutations were first discovered, scientists believed that they occurred more frequently among Jewish women of European descent than women from other groups. As a result, Jewish women of European descent have been more widely tested for *BRCA* mutations than women from other backgrounds. More recently, however, scientists believe that women of some other ethnicities, such as Norwegian, Dutch, and Icelandic, also carry relatively high rates of *BRCA1* and *BRCA2* mutations. Over time, further testing will clarify how prevalent these mutations are in women of different ethnicities.

If you do carry a high-risk *BRCA* mutation, finding out about it lets you take important preventive steps to protect your health:

- You can undergo increased monitoring for breast cancer starting at an earlier age, using tools such as MRI in addition to mammography.
- You can reduce your breast cancer risks by taking steps against DNA damage, including sticking to a healthy diet, avoiding smoking, and getting regular exercise.
- You can choose to take medication that might lower your chances of developing breast cancer. Some research studies have found that giving a breast cancer medication called tamoxifen to healthy women with *BRCA2* mutations lowered their likelihood of developing breast cancer by more than 60 percent. The drug didn't help women with *BRCA1* mutations as much, however. If you carry *BRCA1* or *BRCA2* mutations, talk to your doctor to see if any preventive medications are available to help you.
- You can have surgery to reduce your risk of cancer. For women at greater risk of developing breast cancer, this means undergoing a preventive double mastectomy. This surgery is obviously a huge

decision that isn't undertaken lightly. If you carry a *BRCA1* or *BRCA2* mutation, talk to your doctor and genetic counselor if you are interested in pursuing this step.

- Since women with *BRCA1* and *BRCA2* mutations also have an increased risk of developing ovarian cancer, there are screening, surgical, and medicinal options for ovarian health, as well.

BRCA testing in a family usually starts with a person who has already developed cancer, because it's more likely that if a mutation is present in a family, it will show up in an affected person rather than someone who doesn't have cancer. If the test finds a *BRCA* mutation associated with an increase risk of developing cancer, then other family members can obtain testing for that specific mutation. If you are a member of a family in which there is a known mutation and your test result shows you don't have the mutation, that's usually great news. But even if you don't face any increased inherited risk of breast cancer, you still need to follow general breast cancer screening guidelines.

If you want to learn whether your genome carries any of the more common but less powerful genetic variants related to breast cancer, you can choose to undergo a form of genetic testing that analyzes SNPs related to breast cancer risk. This type of testing is offered by commercial genetic testing companies and is available directly to consumers or through some doctors.

This form of testing does not give you a definitive answer about whether you'll develop breast cancer. If your results show you are at increased risk, however, you can work with your doctor on a plan to reduce your risk. This effort likely includes a focus on a healthy diet, avoiding hormone therapies, and regular breast cancer screenings. It's also important to note that a low risk score is no guarantee of a cancer-free future. Many external factors also increase breast cancer risk, and you'll still need to follow basic preventive steps to reduce your risk and watch for signs of breast cancer. These include undergoing a mammogram every year after the age of 40, monthly self breast exams beginning in your 20s, and regular breast exams conducted by your doctor. Whatever your test shows, it is important to discuss your results with your doctor and a genetic counselor.

Tumor Profiling in Breast Cancer

A growing number of profiles are now available to analyze breast tumors. Many women are already familiar with the most common ones, which focus on hormones, while newer profiles look more deeply at a variety of tumor genes. Breast tumors are now routinely analyzed for their connection with the hormones estrogen and progesterone. Most breast cancers rely on one or both of these hormones to thrive, and are dotted with tiny gene-driven hormone receptors. Some tumors also carry substantial numbers of receptors for HER2, a different growth factor that some cancers need to thrive. By learning your breast tumor's estrogen, progesterone, and HER2 status, you'll get important information about which medications are most likely to help fight your cancer.

Other breast cancer profiles analyze a number of different genes, looking for patterns that reveal the cancer's chances of recurring. This is the type of profile used by Parker Lee, the woman whose story appears at the beginning of this chapter. So far, these profiles are only appropriate for tumors that haven't spread beyond the breast. Many doctors find this new technology interesting, but because clinical trials are currently underway to better define its role in breast cancer treatment, some aren't yet comfortable using it as a basis for treatment decisions. If you have breast cancer that fits the general criteria for one of these profiles, it's worth listening to a variety of opinions before making any treatment decisions based on a tumor analysis. You'll need a doctor's backing to have your tumor profiled, and the usefulness of these profiles varies widely from woman to woman.

Targeted Treatments for Breast Cancer

For some breast cancer treatment decisions, doctors are using information from both standard tumor analysis as well as the specific tumor profiles. One example is Herceptin, which is an ideal choice if your tumor is one of the 25 to 30 percent of breast cancers that tests positive for the growth factor HER2. In cases where Herceptin failed to improve the condition of women with HER2-positive tumors, a newer targeted drug called Tykerb has proven effective at slowing or delaying breast cancer's spread.

If your tumor profile shows that your cancer thrives on the hormones estrogen and progesterone, a group of drugs called aromitase inhibitors can be used to block your cancer's access to them. Tamoxifen was the first such medication used to restrict a breast cancer's hormone supplies, but newer aromitase inhibitors with fewer side effects are becoming increasingly popular choices. In an interesting genetic twist, one scientific team has revealed that about 10 percent of women may not benefit as much from tamoxifen, due to a gene variation that reduced their body's ability to process the drug correctly. Studies are now underway to see if all breast cancer patients should be tested for this gene variation before trying tamoxifen. Doctors are also discovering that breast tumors may change over time, and they are learning how to adjust and switch targeted therapies accordingly.

If your tumor's profile doesn't show that any of these drugs will be effective against your cancer, that information will likely be disappointing. But that answer can also help open other doors. Your doctor may be more willing to offer you experimental treatments if regular medications won't be effective. Experimental advances in breast cancer treatment now arrive regularly in doctors' offices. Ask your doctor about all your profiling and treatment options. You'll still have plenty of treatment choices, even if your tumor profile doesn't offer the answers you were hoping for.

Keep in mind that targeted therapies can't guarantee that your cancer will be cured, or eliminate your need for standard treatments such as chemotherapy or radiation. But if you have breast cancer, take heart in the fact that you have many more treatment options than women did even a decade ago. Gene science is giving breast cancer patients many new reasons for hope.

GENOMICS AND COLORECTAL CANCER

This cancer, which affects the colon, rectum, and other parts of the lower digestive tract, is the third most common cancer in the United States. More than 140,000 new cases are diagnosed each year, and about 55,000 people die from this disease. Since most forms of colorectal cancer grow slowly, many of these deaths would have been prevented by early colon cancer screening, making screening for colorectal cancer an important medical priority.

The role of inherited genetic factors can vary widely. In many cases of the conditions, DNA appears to contribute to risk, but does not emerge as the dominant cause. In these more common forms of the condition, scientists estimate that about 35 percent of risk is genetic.

In about 5 to 10 percent of all colorectal cancer cases, however, mutations with a much stronger effect greatly increase risk. People with these mutations have an 80 to 100 percent chance of developing colorectal cancer during their lifetime. Full cancer profiles for colorectal tumors are still in the process of being developed. But genetic screening for inherited colorectal cancer risk is widely available, as are some targeted drugs.

Risk Testing for Colorectal Cancer

Testing for less common but more powerful genetic factors in colon cancer risk is complex. You'll want to start with your family medical history. Gene experts say you are a good candidate for this form of risk testing if you have a strong family history of the disease, which usually means:

Did You Know ?

If colon cancer is caught early, before it has spread to other organs, the five-year survival rate is 90 percent. But only about 40 percent of all colorectal cancers are caught at this stage, mostly because people don't get screened. Take your doctor's guidelines for colorectal cancer screening seriously, even if you aren't at any increased genetic risk.

• More than one close family member (a parent, sibling, grandparent, or aunt or uncle) who had colorectal cancer.
• A close family member who was diagnosed with colorectal cancer before the age of 50.
• A close family member with a previously diagnosed genetic syndrome that can lead to colorectal cancer.

If colon cancer appears to run in your family, you may be tested for more than one mutation. Several mutations have been directly linked to colorectal cancer. The two most common are:

- Lynch syndrome, also known as Hereditary Nonpolyposis Colorectal Cancer, or HNPCC. Lynch syndrome is linked to about 5 percent of all cases of colorectal cancer, and is caused by mutations in at least four different genes. If you have Lynch syndrome, you have an 80 percent chance of developing colorectal cancer by the age of 75. These mutations also increase your risk of developing other types of cancer, such as endometrial, stomach, or uterine cancer. To make it easier to focus on testing for the right mutations, doctors start by testing the colon tumor.
- Family Adenomatous Polyposis, or FAP. This mutation is much more rare than HNPCC, but it is extremely serious. People with FAP have a 100 percent chance of developing colorectal cancer by the time they turn 45, and in FAP families, some members develop worrisome colon polyps when they are just teenagers. For these reasons, genetic testing and colon scans often begin in FAP families at a young age. FAP is caused by mutations in the *APC* gene, found on Chromosome 5, and is responsible for about 1 percent of all colorectal cancer cases.

If you are found to carry a mutation linked to colorectal cancer, your doctor will offer you one of several treatment options. If you have Lynch syndrome, you'll need frequent colon scans to look for and remove any cancerous growths, or polyps—as often as once a year, often starting in your 40s. You'll also receive frequent exams to check for other types of cancer. If you have an *APC* mutation, doctors recommend beginning colonoscopy in the teens to monitor colon polyps. When these polyps become too numerous to remove each one, doctors recommend removing your entire colon before a serious cancer arises. This is clearly major surgery, and doctors only recommend it because FAP represents such a serious health threat. If you have an *APC* mutation, your doctor and genetic counselor will work with you closely to help you understand your options and what your test results mean for others in your family.

If you are a member of a family in which there is a known mutation and your genetic test results are negative, the news that you don't carry any increased risk of colorectal cancer is probably an enormous relief. But remember that you still share the same risks for the disease as everyone else. To protect your health, continue to follow regular guidelines for colorectal cancer screening. These screenings usually begin at age 50, and include a yearly test to check for blood in your stool—a telltale sign of colorectal cancer—and colon imaging scans at least every five years.

If you want to learn whether your genome carries any of the more common but less powerful genetic variants related to colorectal cancer, you can choose to undergo a form of genetic testing that analyzes SNPs related to colorectal cancer risk. This type of testing is offered by commercial genetic testing companies and is available directly to consumers or through some doctors.

This form of testing does not give you a definitive answer about whether you'll develop colon cancer. If your results show you are at increased risk, however, you can work with your doctor on a plan to reduce your risk. This effort likely includes a focus on a healthy diet, and, most importantly, undergoing regular screenings. It's also important to note that a low risk score is no guarantee of a cancer-free future. Many external factors also increase colorectal cancer risk, and you'll still need to follow basic preventive steps to reduce your risk and watch for signs of colon cancer. Whatever your genetic test shows, it is important to discuss your results with your doctor and a genetic counselor.

Targeted Treatments for Colorectal Cancer

If you have colorectal cancer that is caught early, you'll probably need no additional medicines at all. In early-stage colorectal cancer, surgery to remove any tumors often stops the disease.

But if your cancer has gone unnoticed, and has spread from your digestive tract to other organs, your doctor may offer one or more targeted drugs in addition to surgery, chemotherapy, or radiation. The most promising targeted drug for colorectal cancer is Avastin. As we mentioned earlier in this chapter, Avastin helps control or kill tumors by choking off their blood supply. Some people with aggressive colorectal cancer that has spread to other parts of their body live longer if Avastin is included in their cancer treatment.

If you develop advanced colorectal cancer, Avastin and other targeted drugs can't guarantee your cancer will disappear, but these medicines give you a new array of treatment options. Talk to your doctor about which targeted drugs may be appropriate for your form and stage of cancer.

GENOMICS AND LUNG CANCER

Lung cancer remains the top cause of cancer death in the United States, with more than 170,000 new cases each year and more than 160,000 deaths. In the development of this cancer, your genes play far less of a role than one of your most important health choices—whether or not you smoke. More than 85 percent of lung cancer deaths are linked to smoking. Other factors, including exposure to asbestos and radon, also appear to be a factor in some cases.

Your DNA plays a limited part—scientists estimate about 14 percent of lung cancer risk is genetic. If you want to learn whether your genome carries genetic variants linked to lung cancer risk, you can choose to undergo a form of genetic testing that analyzes SNPs related to lung cancer. This type of testing is offered by commercial genetic testing companies, and is available directly to consumers or through some doctors.

It's important to note, however, that your genetic factors aren't the dominant issue in lung cancer. A lung cancer SNP test does not give you a definitive answer about whether you'll develop this disease. And a low risk score is no guarantee of a cancer-free future. The single best thing you can do to reduce your risk is avoid cigarette smoke and tobacco products. This assertion holds true even if a SNP-based test shows your genetic risk to be relatively low. The toxins in tobacco products are powerful cancer agents, regardless of your genetic factors. Tobacco toxins and carcinogens also harm many other parts of your body, not just your lungs.

Lung cancer comes in two primary forms, characterized by appearance of the cancer cells that make up lung tumors. Small-cell lung cancer, the less common of the two, accounts for about 20 percent of all lung cancer cases. This form of lung cancer usually starts in the larger tubes of the lungs, forming large tumors that grow and spread rapidly.

The other form of lung cancer, called non-small-cell lung cancer, can develop in several different parts of the lungs, such as your smaller breathing tubes or your lungs' mucus glands. Genomic medicine is making gains against this more common form of lung cancer, deploying targeted medications such as Avastin and Tarceva against advanced non-small-cell lung cancer. Tarceva homes in on a tumor protein called epidermal growth factor receptor, or EGFR. This protein helps cancer cells—including lung cancer cells—grow. By blocking EGFR, Tarceva keep some tumors from advancing or spreading.

So far, drugs such as Avastin and Tarceva don't cure lung cancer and don't help every patient who tries them. But the drugs do let some cancer patients live longer, with fewer of the breathing difficulties and other symptoms of advanced lung cancer. Avastin is usually used in combination with chemotherapy, while Tarceva is more likely to be used in patients who don't respond to chemotherapy.

Several large clinical trials are exploring ways to improve our ability to detect lung cancer earlier, when it is easier to treat. Unfortunately, these efforts have yet to yield a consistent, reliable screening method. For now, your best bet against this disease is to limit your risk, primarily by avoiding tobacco smoke.

GENOMICS AND LYMPHOMA

When your body has been battling the flu or another infectious illness, you've probably noticed your lymph nodes. These important parts of your lymphatic system, located at junctures of your body such as your throat and armpits, grow swollen and sore when this important disease-fighting network goes into overdrive to rid your body of disease-causing bacteria or viruses.

When cancer develops in your lymphatic system, the disease is called lymphoma. So far, the causes of lymphoma have proved hard to pin down. Some types of lymphoma appear to have a genetic link, but environmental factors also seem to play a major role in the rise of this cancer.

The term lymphoma covers a variety of lymphatic cancers that divide broadly into two main types—Hodgkin's disease and non-Hodgkin's lymphomas. These two categories reflect how cancer develops differently in various types of lymphatic cells, or lymphocytes. Hodgkin's disease affects a certain subtype of lymphatic cell called a B-lymphocyte. This form of lymphoma is less common, representing about 15 percent of all lymphoma cases.

Non-Hodgkin's lymphomas cover the rest, affecting other subtypes of B-lymphocytes, a different variety of lymphatic cell called a T-lymphocyte, and other aspects of the lymphatic system. With more than 58,000 new cases diagnosed each year, non-Hodgkin's lymphomas are the sixth most common cancer in the United States. There are at least 30 forms of non-Hodgkin's lymphomas, each with a distinct DNA identity, and an exact diagnosis is essential for proper treatment. It's here—in unmasking the exact identity of non-Hodgkin's lymphomas—that genomic medicine has taken its greatest steps against this type of cancer.

Rather than continuing to rely on microscopic analysis and less exact ways of identifying non-Hodgkin's lymphomas, cancer experts have created cancer-profiling tools that distinguish between types of lymphoma more effectively than other diagnostic methods. These profiles make it easier for doctors to pinpoint a lymphoma's identity and choose the most effective medicines. One research study, for example, looked at two forms of non-Hodgkin's lymphoma, one of which requires much more aggressive treatment than the other. If patients with this more virulent form of lymphoma have their disease misdiagnosed, and are given treatment for the less-aggressive form, their survival rate falls from about 80 to 20 percent. Lymphoma profiling was shown to more accurately detect which patients had the more aggressive form of lymphoma and required more intensive treatment. If you have non-Hodgkin's lymphoma, ask your doctor if you are a good candidate for this type of cancer profiling.

Some people with non-Hodgkin's lymphoma are also benefiting from targeted drugs such as Rituxan, which targets about 90 percent of B-cell

Did You Know ?

Lymphoma profiling technology is also helping in the fight against leukemia, which, like lymphoma, is a major form of blood cancer. About 35,000 people are diagnosed with leukemia in the United States each year. Also like lymphoma, the disease comes in several sub-types, each requiring specific treatment. Scientists in the United States and Europe are now working to make cancer profiles similar to those used against lymphoma a standard part of leukemia care.

lymphomas. When used together with chemotherapy, Rituxan improves a person's chances of survival by as much as 47 percent. Rituxan is fully approved for use in many cases of B-cell lymphoma.

GENOMICS AND OVARIAN CANCER

Ovarian cancer is the seventh most common form of cancer among women in the United States, affecting more than 20,000 women a year. But it is the fourth most deadly cancer among women, killing about 15,000 women a year. This is due, in large part, to the fact that ovarian cancer is difficult to detect until it is advanced and has spread to other organs. For most women, the lifetime risk of developing ovarian cancer is very low—a little over 1 percent. But for women with mutations in their *BRCA1* or *BRCA2* genes, the same mutations linked to an increased risk of breast cancer, that risk is much higher, between 15 percent and 50 percent.

BRCA mutations are believed to play a role in about 5 to 10 percent of ovarian cancer cases. If a close relative, such as your mother, grandmother, aunts, or sisters, has developed breast or ovarian cancer, especially at a relatively young age, turn to the section on *BRCA* genetic testing for breast cancer risk earlier in this chapter. The same general testing guidelines and considerations apply to both breast and ovarian cancer risk. If your family background matches that of women with known *BRCA* mutations, you may want to consider genetic testing.

If your *BRCA* test results point to an increased risk of ovarian cancer, your doctor and genetic counselor will talk to you about a variety of medical options, including preventive removal of your ovaries. This surgery, called an oophorectomy, reduces your risk of ovarian cancer by 95 percent. For women with *BRCA2* mutations who haven't yet gone through menopause, this surgery also reduces the risk of breast cancer by about 50 percent.

While this surgery can protect you against cancer, it's also a major medical decision. If you haven't yet gone through menopause, removing your ovaries leads to the loss of your female hormones, putting you into early menopause. Most cancer centers suggest the use of hormone replacement therapy until age 50 if the ovaries are removed before that age. Some younger women with *BRCA* mutations prefer to receive frequent cancer screening instead of undergoing this surgery, although it is not clear that the screening is effective. For others, removing most of their risk of cancer is paramount. Your doctor and genetic counselor can help you decide which options are right for you.

If your *BRCA* test results are negative, that's great news. But remember that even if you don't carry an increased risk of ovarian cancer, you still share the same overall risks as the general population. Make sure to get regular check-ups, especially if you are over 50, and talk to your doctor if you have persistent symptoms such as abdominal bloating, abdominal discomfort, persistent fatigue, or unexplained weight gain or loss.

GENOMICS AND PROSTATE CANCER

Prostate cancer is the most common cancer among men in the United States, with more than 230,000 new cases diagnosed each year. It is the fourth most common cause of cancer deaths among men, killing about 27,000 men each year.

A man's age represents his highest risk factor for prostate cancer. The disease is rare in men younger than 45, and most cases are found in men who are over 65. Most men have about a 14 percent chance of developing prostate cancer by the time they are 80 years old. But family history and race also play a role, indicating that genetic factors affect prostate cancer as well. Scientists estimate that a little more than 40 percent of prostate cancer risk is genetic. If you are a man with a father, son, or brother with prostate cancer, scientists believe your own risk of developing prostate cancer is two to three times higher than average. African-American and Caucasian men in the United States develop prostate cancer more often than men from other ethnic backgrounds, and African-American men with prostate cancer are more likely to die from their disease than men from other groups.

If you want to learn whether you carry any genetic variants related to prostate cancer, you can choose to undergo a form of genetic testing that analyzes SNPs related to prostate cancer risk. This type of testing is offered by commercial genetic testing companies, and is available directly to consumers or through some doctors.

This form of testing does not give you a definitive answer about whether you'll develop prostate cancer. If your results show you are at increased risk, however, you can work with your doctor on a plan to reduce your risk. This effort likely includes a focus on a healthy diet, and regular screenings.

It's also important to note that a low risk score is no guarantee of a cancer-free future. In African-American men, these tests may underestimate prostate cancer risk. Many external factors also increase prostate cancer risk, and you'll still need to follow basic preventive steps to reduce your risk and watch for signs of prostate cancer. If you are 50 or older, you should have a PSA blood test and physical exam to check for prostate cancer each year. If you are African-American, or have a strong family history of prostate cancer, you should begin this testing at age 45. Men with very

African-Americans Need to Pay Special Attention to Prostate Cancer

African-American men with prostate cancer are two to three more times likely to die from their disease than men from other backgrounds. The reasons for this aren't yet well understood. Genetic factors, more limited access to medical care, or lifestyle influences such as diet may all play a role. If you are African-American, follow your doctor's recommendations on prostate cancer screening closely, especially if someone else in your family has had prostate cancer.

strong family histories of prostate cancer, in which several of your close relatives developed prostate cancer at an early age, are urged to start these tests at age 40.

FREQUENTLY ASKED QUESTIONS ABOUT CANCER AND GENOMICS

Q. I'm finding it hard to see exactly how genomic advances against cancer really count as good news. Overall, the number of new cancer cases each year seems to keep going up. I hear about friends and coworkers diagnosed with cancer all the time. With numbers like that, how can gene science really be making much of a difference?

A. It's true that, overall, total cases of new cancer in the United States generally keep increasing. But a good part of this climb isn't due to any major medical failure in the fight against cancer. Instead, the numbers reflect the fact that more Americans are getting older. Everyone's risk of cancer increases with age, so it makes sense that as the population grows grayer, total cancer cases will go up. The good news is that genomics is brightening the prospects for many of these new cancer patients, giving them better chances for beating their disease. Doctors once had fewer options for treating cancer, making a cancer diagnosis a death sentence for many people. Now, more people with cancer are surviving than ever before.

Q. There is a lot of conflicting information on chemicals and cancer. On one hand, I keep hearing that certain chemicals can cause cancer, and that even everyday household cleaners and/or plastics can't be trusted. But then some expert will say that's it all about genetics, or that it's not clear how much of a particular chemical will make you sick or give you cancer. If some chemicals cause cancer, why can't anyone figure out exactly how much of them we can tolerate in the first place?

A. It can be frustrating and frightening to hear that a common substance is bad for you, but not know exactly how much of it you need to watch out for. This uncertainty exists because, until recently, there was no easy way to test these risks. It wouldn't be acceptable to experiment with chemicals on people to see which levels are safe and which are dangerous. But a new field of health science called biomonitoring, hopes to fill in this gap. In biomonitoring, people's blood and bodies are measured for risky substances, and their health is tracked over a long period of time to see what effects these substances may have. California has launched a statewide biomonitoring program, and other states are likely to follow suit. Over time, biomonitoring should provide more answers on the danger levels and health effects of many of the chemicals that surround us.

Q. *My dad has smoked for most of his life and has never gotten lung cancer. I smoke too, and my doctor keeps telling me to quit. But if your genes can increase or decrease your risk of cancer, maybe we've got some built-in barrier against lung cancer? If my dad smokes two packs a day and doesn't have lung cancer, isn't there a decent chance I have some genetic protection against it?*

A. That kind of assumption puts your health at enormous risk. In some people, genes do affect their susceptibility to cancer. But most cases of cancer have little to do with inherited strengths or risks. Most cancers arise when outside factors—like toxic chemicals in cigarette smoke—damage a person's DNA. Relatively little is known about inherited susceptibility to lung cancer, but a great deal is known about how cigarette smoke causes cancer, not just in the lungs, but in other parts of the body, as well. You can cut your family's risk of cancer enormously right now by throwing away your cigarettes, and convincing your dad to do the same.

Q. *I'm a young woman with lots of ovarian cancer in my family. My grandmother had ovarian cancer, as did both her daughters (my aunts). But all these relatives are on my dad's side of the family. Ovarian cancer seems like a woman's issue, so am I at less risk because these cases appear on my dad's side of the family tree?*

A. Even though your family's cancer is on your dad's side, you may still face increased risk. If a cancer-related mutation runs in your father's family, your dad may have inherited it from his mother. As a man, he won't develop ovarian cancer, but he could still have passed the mutation on to you. Gene experts take the medical history of both sides of the family into account when assessing ovarian or breast cancer risk. You should talk with a genetic counselor about your family history. Genetic testing, either for you or relatives on your father's side of the family, may be an option worth considering.

Q. *My grandfather has lymphoma, and his doctor wants him to enroll in a special study that will provide a detailed profile of his cancer. I know we should be excited about this opportunity, but we're actually kind of scared. What if the profile delivers bad news? What if it says my grandfather's cancer is aggressive and hard to treat, or that he'll die in six months no matter what we do? My grandfather is frail, and his cancer care is exhausting. We're afraid that if he gets a bad report, he'll just give up entirely.*

A. Your concerns about your grandfather's profile are completely legitimate. Cancer profiles offer a wealth of useful medical information, but in a few cases, they can also be double-edged swords. If the profile says that the cancer may be responsive to a particular drug or requires a very precise type of treatment, that information is invaluable. If the profile says that your grandfather's cancer is hard to treat, that tough news might carry a silver lining. It could allow your grandfather and his doctors to consider experimental therapies more readily. The information could also allow your grandfather and his caregivers to make a decision against any further exhausting treatments. An entirely different cancer specialty, called palliative care, helps some patients who are dying to do so in comfort and with dignity. And remember, this choice ultimately rests with your grandfather. Cancer profiling is usually a patient's choice, not a requirement. No one can force him into a cancer profile if he just isn't emotionally ready.

Q. *I just found out that I have invasive breast cancer, and targeted drugs like Herceptin sound like a great option. But my doctor still wants me to undergo surgery and chemotherapy and radiation—all choices that scare me just as much as the cancer. Why can't I just use targeted drugs and spare my body a lot of trauma?*

A. Targeted medicines do offer new hope in the fight against cancer, and many doctors think these drugs represent the future of cancer treatment. But right now, they also have to face the fact that these drugs are new, and don't provide a complete set of weapons against this disease. Targeted drugs also don't work against every form of a particular cancer. Herceptin, for example, is a good fit for only 25 to 30 percent of breast cancer patients. Your doctor is offering you options with proven track records against your type of breast cancer. If you aren't sure about those treatments, seek second or even third opinions. While you aren't likely to find a breast cancer specialist who only recommends using targeted drugs at this time, you may find reassurance in hearing a variety of medical perspectives and choices.

KEEP IN MIND

As you consider making genomics part of your plans for cancer prevention or cancer care, here are a few key points to help you along the way.

Cancer is essentially a disease of damaged DNA that causes certain cells to grow out of control. But while genes drive cancer, most cases of cancer are not inherited. Instead, harmful external effects such as toxic chemicals or radiation usually cause the DNA damage that leads to cancer.

Genomic science, working to unravel the workings of this disease, is creating a powerful new understanding of cancer. Doctors now know, for example, that illnesses we've long lumped together as breast cancer or lymphoma actually come in many distinct sub-types, each with different features and weaknesses.

This improved knowledge of cancer is also offering new tools to fight it. Genetic tests can now reveal SNPs and mutations that increase some people's risk of certain cancers. Gene scans provide detailed profiles of tumors that reveal their exact identities, habits, and vulnerabilities. Increasingly, doctors can use specific features of tumors to choose targeted treatments well designed to control or kill particular cancers.

If you're wondering if you've inherited an increased risk of cancer, take a close look at your family medical history. Inherited cancer risk appears most frequently in families with multiple cases of cancer in several generations, some diagnosed at a relatively young age. Discuss your concerns with your doctor or a genetic counselor. If you are interested in genetic testing for inherited cancer risk, pursue this testing through your doctor and genetic counselor if at all possible. If you must use a direct-to-consumer test, purchase one from a company that offers the services of licensed genetic counselors. These test results can be difficult to understand and are so important to your health that they deserve an expert's attention.

Given that most cases of cancer arise from acquired mutations, your best bet for lowering your risk of cancer is to help protect your DNA from damage. Avoid influences known to harm genes and trigger cancer, such as excessive ultraviolet radiation from the sun or tanning salons or the toxins in cigarette smoke. You can also boost your DNA's ability to repair itself by keeping yourself healthy; get regular exercise and follow a diet high in brightly colored fruits and vegetables.

Cancer remains a frightening fact of modern life. But genomic science is making great strides against this illness, and many doctors say genomic approaches to cancer hold the key to fighting it. Genomic insights first developed against cancer are also helping improve knowledge and treatments in other important aspects of your health. Chapter 6 looks at one of these critical areas—the health of your blood and your heart.

CHAPTER SIX

YOUR GENES, HEALTHY BLOOD AND A HEALTHY HEART

Scattered all over the country, the eight children in the Roberts family joked that they single-handedly kept the telephone company afloat. All grown, with kids of their own, the five brothers and three sisters stayed in touch by spending hours on the phone each week, laughing their way through raucous family conference calls.

One Sunday, a couple of hours before a planned family call, Sam Roberts took a few minutes to chop some logs into firewood in his Pennsylvania backyard. The September day was unseasonably hot, and the wood hard and knotty. Sam, 38 and in excellent shape, found that his chore had turned into a tough workout.

Suddenly, his wife Hannah heard the axe fall with a thud. She looked out the window to see Sam lying on the ground. He had passed out, and when she raced to his side, she couldn't find a pulse. Hannah frantically called 911 and started CPR, but Sam died in her arms before the ambulance arrived.

Reeling from shock, Hannah realized Sam's family call was just about to start. She dialed into the group number, and found two of his brothers, Josh and Evan, already on the line. Tears rolling down her face, Hannah told them what had happened. Josh started asking a thousand questions. Evan, 34, uttered only "What?! What?" before his end of the line suddenly fell silent.

It took the rest of the family another hour to learn that Evan died that day, too, collapsing after hearing the news about Sam. His heart had also stopped, and paramedics who rushed to his home couldn't revive him.

The surviving brothers and sisters, grieving and worried, started trying to figure out what had happened that day. Four went to talk to their doctors, explaining the two brothers' deaths. Their mother had suffered several bad fainting spells when she was young, but no one had ever thought her blackouts added up to anything more than occasional dizziness. Three of the doctors measured blood pressure, pulse, and heartbeat. Each result seemed fine, so they told the siblings that Sam and Evan's deaths were probably a tragic coincidence.

Josh's doctor, however, heard the story and immediately sent him to a heart specialist skilled in genetics. That specialist put Josh through a series of sophisticated heart tests, including one that simulated the effects of shock or hard exercise. Josh's heart rhythm suddenly shot out of control. The test, followed by a genetic analysis, revealed that he had inherited a dangerous mutation that ran in the family. The mutation makes some of the Roberts' hearts prone to beating wildly and stopping under duress. They had probably inherited the mutation from their mother, whose gene variant had made her black out, but luckily never killed her. Five of the eight Roberts children proved to have the gene variant, and some of their children did, as well. By taking steps to control their heart rhythm with medication or implanted defibrillators, the surviving children and their families have since avoided any repeats of that terrible September day.

Thanks to genomic medicine, people like the Roberts children are increasingly able to understand what really lies behind heart problems that have long seemed to run in the family. Some are uncovering the causes of previously unexplained deaths. Others are gaining new insights into less dramatic but equally important issues related to a healthy heart, including risks for high cholesterol, excessive levels of iron in their blood, or a heart attack. Thanks to a gene test, some are now even able to receive the most appropriate dose of a common medication that helps prevent blood clots. With heart disease a major public health problem in the United States, responsible for every one in three deaths, genomic advances in cardiac care are already saving lives.

This chapter takes a look at just some of the ways genomic care is transforming the world of heart health. Some advances made in rare diseases of the heart offer important insights into more common conditions. Others are changing your medical options for keeping your heart and blood healthy, especially controlling your cholesterol and preventing dangerous blood clots.

Understanding how your genes can help you keep your heart healthy, however, requires knowing a few basics about your heart and the blood it pumps. We begin with a quick look at the main pieces of this essential system.

YOUR HEART, BLOOD AND THE DELIVERY SYSTEM

Every part of your body needs a few essentials to keep going—oxygen from the air you breathe, water from the fluids you drink, and nutrients from your food. And every part of your body is able to enjoy those essentials thanks to your blood, a liquid transportation system that delivers these necessities everywhere, from your brain to a tiny cell helping to grow a new nail at the end of your big toe. Nutrients and water flow in the blood. Oxygen gets toted by your red blood cells, which give your blood its distinctive color and literally keep your cells breathing by bringing them oxygen and hauling away waste gas.

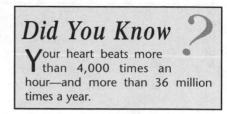

Your blood does all this traveling thanks to your heart, that powerhouse pump in the middle of your chest. Each heartbeat pushes blood throughout your body. Oxygen-rich blood leaves your heart through a system of blood vessels called arteries, while depleted blood returns for refueling through vessels called veins. Your arteries dispense blood rich in oxygen and important nutrients to every part of your body—including your heart, which needs lots of fuel to drive all the work it does. This entire network is called your cardiovascular system, encompassing the heart and all the vessels connected to it.

As indispensable delivery chutes, your arteries do their job best when they run clean and clear. They have a protective lining, which lets blood flow freely when the lining is thin and smooth. If that lining gets damaged, however, your delivery system starts to bog down. The pressure of the blood flowing through your arteries might be too high, tearing a tiny hole in the lining. Dangerous chemicals from cigarette smoke, high levels of sugar in your blood, or any number of other irritants might do similar damage, making the lining inflamed. Your body will try to fix the damage by ordering your blood to use cholesterol, a waxy blood-borne fat, to plug the spot.

That patching system sounds like a good idea, but it doesn't always work as intended. If you have too much of a particularly sticky type of

The Blood Pressure Gene

High blood pressure, or hypertension—a condition in which your blood pushes against the walls of your arteries too forcefully—affects nearly 1 in 3 American adults. It's a serious and often silent problem, sometimes going undetected until it causes heart trouble, a stroke, or kidney failure. Stress, diet, and alcohol all affect blood pressure, but doctors have long realized that two other factors with clear gene links also play a part—family history and race.

Now, two research efforts are making headway in understanding the genomics of high blood pressure. The first endeavor, the Family Blood Pressure Program, studied the DNA of about 18,000 Americans from different regions and ethnic backgrounds to start finding genes related to high blood pressure and see how they might help in treating this common illness. Another team of scientists is working to develop a genetic test to reveal if a person faces an increased risk from eating foods with high levels of salt—a nutrient often linked to high blood pressure.

Genes Related to Strokes

As genomic science works to pinpoint genes linked to heart disease, information on one cardiac-related condition has lagged a little behind: stroke. Strokes, caused by either a blocked or ruptured blood vessel that feeds the brain, are a major cause of death and disability. About 700,000 Americans have a stroke each year.

The blocked blood vessels that give rise to many strokes are somewhat similar to those found in coronary artery disease, often clogged by the narrowed, inflamed arterial buildups that are the mark of atherosclerosis. Strokes also carry many medical complexities all their own, making specific stroke-related genes difficult to pinpoint. For example, a team of scientists announced that a particular variant of a gene on Chromosome 5 called *PDE4D* increases a person's risk of stroke anywhere from three to five times. But because it remains unclear exactly how *PDE4D* affects stroke risk, genetic tests or related treatments remain out of reach for now.

cholesterol in your blood called low density lipoprotein (LDL), the arterial plug can get too big. Your body may try to smooth it out, but sometimes that doesn't work, or it only increases inflammation in the area. Another component of your blood, sensing trouble, tries to help by building a clot over the damaged spot. Often, though, that only leads to a bigger problem—an inflamed tangle of cholesterol and clot. If this plug grows large enough, it can badly restrict an artery's flow, or block it entirely. And if the clot breaks free, it can travel through your blood to clog other arteries. If one of these blockages narrows an artery that feeds your heart, the resulting condition is called coronary artery disease—literally an illness of the blood vessels nourishing the heart. This can starve your heart muscle and cause a heart attack. If a clot or plug blocks an artery to your brain, it can bring on a stroke.

Many of the factors that shape the health of your blood, heart, and arteries are in your hands. You choose most of what goes into your blood—your food, your beverages, and other ingredients such as cigarette smoke—and have plenty of say over keeping oxygen flowing to your cells, your heart pumping, and your arteries clear. But your genes also shape this system. Some people may have gene features that don't let them deliver oxygen as efficiently. A few have hearts with structural or functional defects that don't have normal power or efficiency. Other people carry genes that don't let them handle cholesterol well, boosting their risk of plugged arteries, heart attacks, strokes, and even sudden cardiac arrest.

To see some of these genes at work, we take a look at some of the more common gene-linked cardiovascular conditions. Thousands of genes affect your blood, blood vessels, and heart, and not every gene's function is clear yet. But where genes' roles have been clearly defined, you now have the chance to use your DNA to help keep your heart and blood healthy. Let's start with gene variants that hamper the blood's ability to do one of its most essential jobs—deliver oxygen.

ANEMIA

Circulating throughout your body, your red blood cells are some of your body's hardest-working—and essential—porters. These cells carry oxygen to your cells, and tote away wastes for removal. Just one drop of human blood contains more than 4 million red blood cells, and they are so essential for good health that your body constantly makes new ones to keep those numbers so high. Some people, however, have blood that can't transport oxygen well. They may have fewer red blood cells than normal. Others have red blood cells that are lacking in hemoglobin, the component of the cell that carries the oxygen. Either problem gives rise to anemia, an illness marked by the body's inability to deliver oxygen effectively.

You've probably heard of anemia, as it's a very common condition. Most of the time, it's a relatively mild problem caused by poor diet, and is easy to cure with higher consumption of iron—which helps you make hemoglobin—or other important nutrients. But some people with anemia can pin the problem on their genes. Some mutations can lead to serious forms of anemia that can be painful or even deadly. Here, we look at two of the more common inherited anemias—sickle cell anemia and beta thalassemia.

How Genes Are Involved

Both sickle cell anemia and beta thalassemia arise from different mutations in the *HBB* gene, found on Chromosome 11. The *HBB* gene provides instructions for making an essential part of hemoglobin, and mutations anywhere in this gene can lead to problems with oxygen delivery.

The *HBB* mutation responsible for sickle cell anemia distorts the shape of red blood cells, twisting them from their normal round form into a crescent, or sickle, shape. These misshapen cells die more quickly than normal ones, creating a shortage of red blood cells. They can also block small blood vessels, causing severe pain and organ damage. This condition is inherited in an autosomal recessive manner, so a person must inherit two copies of this *HBB* mutation to develop sickle cell disease.

Sickle cell anemia is one of the more common inherited blood disorders in the United States, appearing most often in African-Americans. About eight percent of African-Americans are sickle cell carriers—that is, they have a single mutation. Carriers rarely have health problems. But sickle cell anemia is not limited to African-Americans; people of other ethnic backgrounds may carry the mutation and develop the disease as well. In general, it appears more often in people whose ancestors have historically lived in Africa, Mediterranean countries, the Arabian peninsula, India, and parts of South and Central America. Among Latinos, one in every 1,000 to 1,400 people develops sickle cell disease.

The *HBB* mutations responsible for beta thalassemia either reduce or eliminate the amount of hemoglobin in a person's red blood cells. More than 200 mutations related to beta thalassemia have been discovered, and some create more serious health problems than others. The most serious form of beta thalassemia, called beta thalassemia major, starts causing severe health problems in the first two years of a child's life, robbing an infant or toddler of energy, stunting growth, and damaging vital organs such as the liver and heart. Without proper treatment, most people with beta thalassemia major die at a young age. A person must usually inherit two copies of a beta thalassemia mutation to fall ill, although carriers may sometimes develop a milder form of anemia.

Like sickle cell anemia, beta thalassemia mutations follow a geographic pattern, occurring most often in people from Mediterranean countries, North Africa, the Middle East, the Indian subcontinent, and Southeast Asia. While carrier rates vary from region to region, they can be quite high. On the Mediterranean island of Cyprus, for example, one in every seven people is a beta thalassemia carrier. While beta thalassemia occurs at lower rates in the United States, it affects more than 300,000 people around the globe. (For more information on a program to reduce the rate of thalassemia on Cyprus, see Chapter 3.)

It's important to note that while these and other inherited anemias go by different names, they also sometimes affect or enhance each other. Each of the mutations behind these conditions affects a critical aspect of your blood, and if a person inherits multiple anemia-related mutations, they may develop especially challenging forms of anemia. For example, a baby may have one parent who carries one sickle cell mutation and another who carries one thalassemia mutation. While each parent may have healthy blood, the baby may develop a serious illness. Carrier testing and newborn screening are both available for anemia-related mutations and illnesses. If you come from an ethnic group more prone to inherited anemias, it's important to consider carrier testing before starting a family. It's also important to have your newborn baby undergo newborn screening. For more information on these tests, see Chapter 3.

It's likely that genes also play a role in more common, less serious forms of anemia, making some people more susceptible to developing the condition as a result of their diet. For now, though, genomic scientists are still investigating the identities and functions of these genes.

Did You Know **?**

Sickle cell anemia and beta thalassemia are terrible diseases, but their mutations probably became significant in some parts of the world because they helped the body's efforts to stop a different illness—malaria.

Malaria is a dangerous, sometimes fatal sickness carried by mosquitoes, which infect a person's blood with the malaria parasite when they bite. Malaria is usually found in the same regions where sickle cell and thalassemia mutations were historically more common. Scientists have found that people with one copy of one of these mutations are more likely to survive acute malaria infection, because their hemoglobin makes it harder for malaria to take hold in their blood. It's only when someone has two copies of one of these mutations that this natural defense morphs into an entirely different illness.

Genetic Testing for Inherited Anemia

Genetic tests for both sickle cell anemia and beta thalassemia are readily available through doctors. Given the complex mutations these tests must track, along with the serious health problems that accompany them, direct-to-consumer genetics companies are much less likely to offer these tests.

If you are healthy, but come from an ethnic background with more frequent appearances of inherited anemias, you also have the opportunity to find out whether you carry an anemia-related mutation. This form of testing, called carrier testing, helps determine your risk of having a child with inherited anemia. If you are thinking about having children and want to know more about the conditions your child could potentially inherit, talk to your doctor about undergoing carrier testing. In situations when a couple is already pregnant, and both partners are found to be carriers, prenatal genetic testing can reveal whether a developing baby has inherited any anemia-related mutations. (For more information on carrier and prenatal testing, see Chapter 3.)

Special Considerations for Inherited Anemias

Many African-Americans are of mixed heritage, carrying a blend of African, Caucasian, and Native American ancestry. The same is true of Latinos from Caribbean and Central or South American countries with large populations of African descent. If you are an African-American or Latino of mixed race, your varied ancestry offers a great deal of protection against inheriting two copies of a sickle cell mutation and developing sickle cell disease. But it doesn't prevent you from being a carrier. Even if you are of mixed race, your doctor will likely offer you sickle cell carrier testing if you are pregnant or considering having children.

In the United States, carrier testing for thalassemia has historically been offered most often to people of Mediterranean or Southeast Asian descent. But emerging genetic research shows that carrier rates for thalassemia are also high among people from the Middle East and Indian subcontinent. In Iran, for example, beta thalassemia is the most common genetic illness, and in some parts of the country more than 10 percent of the population carries a mutation. If your family or ancestors come from these regions, take the initiative to talk to your doctor about carrier testing.

How You Can Treat Inherited Anemias

Sickle cell anemia, beta thalassemia, and most other forms of genetic anemia are serious illnesses requiring specialty care. While there is still no way to repair or override the *HBB* mutations causing these illnesses, medical treatments to ease their effects have improved.

Sickle cell disease, for example, requires constant medical therapy, including folic acid supplements to boost red blood cell production. Some patients require blood transfusions, and others need strong pain medication and other medical help when blocked blood vessels damage tissues, triggering episodes called sickle cell crises. These bouts of sickle cell crisis often bring severe pain to the abdomen, joints, chest, or the large bones of the body, such as those in the legs and arms. Sickle cell crises can also block blood flow to important parts of a person's immune system, raising the risk of infection. While the disease remains difficult to manage, better treatments have improved prospects for many sickle cell patients. In the past, many people with sickle cell disease died of organ failure before the age of 40. Now, many are living into their 50s and 60s. Beta thalassemia also requires constant treatment, including red blood cell transfusions every two to three weeks to keep a person's hemoglobin levels sufficiently high. This large number of transfusions creates its own set of difficult medical complications, but still, these treatments allow many people with beta thalassemia to live well into adulthood.

The Bottom Line on Inherited Anemias

These forms of anemia are far less common, but far more serious, than the diet-related anemia that many people experience. If you come from an ethnic background with higher rates of inherited anemia, talk to your doctor about genetic testing, even if you are healthy. By learning whether you carry a mutation linked to inherited anemia, you can better understand the risks to any children you may have, and reveal risks that other members of your family may have as well.

BLOOD CLOTTING DISORDERS

Your blood's ability to clot is a vital part of your self-defense system. When blood vessels are injured, tiny cells called platelets receive signals to lump together and plug the damaged area. Helped by the activity of proteins called clotting factor, this lump becomes a protective cover that stops blood loss and allows the damaged area to heal.

In some people, however, blood clots don't form normally. Some people have an increased tendency to form blood clots, a condition called thrombophilia. These clots, also called thromboses, can break free from the blood vessels where they first form and travel through the blood stream, blocking arteries and sometimes harming the heart or lungs. One form of thrombophilia, called deep vein thrombosis, or DVT, is an especially pressing medical concern. These clots form in large interior veins, often in the thigh or calf, and if they move elsewhere in the body, can cause serious lung damage or even death. According to estimates by the American Heart Association, about 300,000 Americans develop deep vein thrombosis each year. Here are some of the reasons why:

- Doctors now perform hundreds of thousands of hip- and knee-replacement surgeries each year, and people undergoing these procedures have been shown to face a higher risk of DVT.

- Extended periods of sitting, such as during long airplane or car travel, increase a person's risk of DVT.
- Some women may also be at increased risk if they take birth control pills.

Genetic factors, however, can further increase these risks, as well as create unique risks of their own.

How Genes Are Involved

While many cases of thrombophilia can be linked to external factors, genomic scientists have revealed that about 50 percent of a person's risk is genetic. Several genes have been linked to thrombophilia; the two most common are Factor V Leiden and prothrombin mutations:

- Factor V Leiden is the most common form of inherited thrombophilia. Factor V Leiden mutations arise on the *F5* gene, located on Chromosome 1. The *F5* gene is critical to blood clot formation, and people with the Factor V Leiden mutation are prone to a blood-clotting process that continues longer than normal. According to federal health estimates, about 3 to 8 percent of the Caucasian population in the United States carries one copy of the mutation, and 1 in every 5,000 people has two copies. A single copy increases a person's risk of developing a blood clot anywhere from four to eight times, and two copies increase a person's risk about 80 times. The Factor V Leiden mutation is less common in other ethnic groups.
- The prothrombin mutation arises on the prothrombin gene, located on Chromosome 11. This gene carries the code for an important piece of the blood clotting process. About 1 to 2 percent of the

"Economy Class" Syndrome — It's More About Genes Than Price

Deep vein thrombosis has gotten plenty of press over worries that it's more likely to hit people who fly long distances frequently, especially business travelers who shuttle around the country in cramped airplane cabins. But the condition has nothing to do with the price—or luxury—of your airplane seat. If you travel long distances frequently, either by plane or car, your best strategy to avoid a deep vein clot is to get up and move around every hour or two, and do small exercises that keep the blood flowing in your legs and calves. Many airlines now include descriptions of these exercises in their in-flight magazines.

Staying active while traveling is especially important if you have a family history of blood clots or thrombophilia mutations. If you are aware of any genetic risks, and make sure you keep your blood moving while you travel, you can go a long way toward avoiding a blood clot, whether you're flying in roomier first-class luxury or in crowded economy seating.

Caucasian population carries one copy of the mutation. Carrying one copy increases a person's risk of blood clots two to three times. Having two copies of the mutation is much more rare, and while two copies do increase a person's risks of blood clots further, exactly how much that risk increases isn't yet clear. Other ethnic groups have lower rates of the prothrombin mutation.

Genetic Testing for Blood Clotting Disorders

Gene tests for Factor V Leiden and prothrombin mutations are now widely available through both established medical networks and direct-to-consumer genetic testing companies. Doctors usually recommend that you talk with a medical professional or genetic counselor before deciding on testing, and obtain your test through your physician.

The Royal Disease

A genetic tendency to form blood clots may be relatively common, but it's more likely you've heard of the opposite—a genetic inability to form clots when needed. This condition, called hemophilia, is rare. But it has a famous place in history, and it has helped open new doors in genetic medicine.

Hemophilia's notoriety arises from its appearance in the royal descendants of the British monarch Queen Victoria in the 19th and 20th centuries, rewriting the political map of Europe as it spread through royal bloodlines and contributing to the overthrow of the Romanovs, the last royal family of imperial Russia. One of Queen Victoria's sons had hemophilia, and two of her daughters were carriers. One daughter eventually passed the disease to Victoria's great-grandson Alexei Romanov, the young prince born as the last intended heir of the Russian throne. The story of Alexei and his family—including how the Romanovs struggled to help the suffering boy and their eventual execution by the revolutionary forces that gave rise to the Soviet Union—has left many people with the impression that hemophilia is primarily a European or Russian illness. This is not the case, however; hemophilia occurs in all races and ethnic groups.

The disease has two forms, each caused by a different gene on the X chromosome. Hemophilia's connection to the X chromosome makes it a sex-linked recessive disorder, meaning that men, who carry only one copy of the X chromosome, have no healthy X to protect them if they inherit the hemophilia mutation. Women, who carry two copies of the X, are far less likely to develop the disease because they are likely to inherit one healthy X that can shield them from a risk-related one. As a result, almost all cases of hemophilia arise in males, often starting in infancy or childhood. (For more information on sex-linked disorders, see Chapter 1.)

About 18,000 people have hemophilia in the United States, and about 400 babies are born with it each year. Treating hemophilia is extremely complicated, involving a blend of pain-relief and injected medicines that help the blood to clot. It's essential for hemophiliacs to avoid injury, but even after taking extra cautions, many people with hemophilia still experience sporadic episodes of dangerous internal bleeding.

Hemophilia is now a key focus of research into gene therapy, as scientists look for a way to fix or override the mutations that cause this devastating disease. Gene therapy is discussed in Chapter 9.

If you choose a direct-to-consumer test, however, you have several important issues to consider. The first is cost. Such tests are usually offered in a package deal that analyzes two or more genes related to thrombophilia, or it looks at your risk for thrombophilia alongside many other conditions. These combination tests may cost at least several hundred dollars, and they usually aren't covered by insurance.

It's also important to note that genetic testing for Factor V Leiden and prothrombin usually isn't recommended for the general population. Factor V Leiden mutations occur in up to eight percent of Caucasians in the United States—meaning that more than 90 percent of this population group is mutation-free. In other ethnic groups, even fewer have a mutation. Overall, your risk of thrombophilia-related mutations is very low, and a genetic test isn't necessary for most people. However, if you have a family history of blood clots, or if you have already developed a clot and want to help your relatives understand their own risks, it may be more worthwhile to test these genes.

If you do pursue testing, keep in mind that a positive test result doesn't mean you'll definitely develop blood clots. A positive result only means you face greater risk. If you receive a positive test result, be sure to talk to a genetic counselor or your doctor, who can help you develop a plan to reduce your risk of blood clots.

Special Considerations for Blood Clotting Disorders

Your family medical history is one of your best indicators of your risk of thrombophilia. Signs of a family propensity toward blood clots include:

RED FLAG!

Which Blood Clotting Test Is Right for You?

If you are interested in a direct-to-consumer genetic test for increased blood-clot risk, you may find that your available options are more complicated than you expect. Companies that offer these tests often feature two different options: one big gene test "package" that looks for two or more mutations related to thrombophilia or a menu of separate tests.

If you know a particular mutation has already been found in your family, that makes your choice easy. You can pick a test for the same mutation to see if you share your relatives' increased blood clot risk. But if you aren't sure which, if any, mutation you might be at risk for, it can be hard to know where to start. And with these tests costing hundreds of dollars, you probably don't want to choose tests at random.

Before you spend any money, your best bet is to get an informed perspective. Reliable direct-to-consumer testing companies offer the services of genetic counselors. Contact the company and ask to speak with a counselor before you pick any particular test. You can also talk to your doctor, or ask for a referral to a genetic counselor. Since most people's risks for thrombophilia genes are already low, and tests for these genes take a big bite out of your wallet, an outside opinion can help you make the best choice.

- Relatives who have had strokes.
- Relatives who have had blood clots or are taking blood-thinning medication.
- Female relatives who have had second trimester miscarriages.

If blood clots run in your family, genetic testing is a more worthwhile option. Even if you haven't had a genetic test, let your doctor know about your family history, especially before undergoing surgery. If there is time before the surgery, your surgical team may consider genetic testing or give you blood-thinning medication to reduce your risk of clots after your operation.

If you are a woman with a family history of thrombophilia and are either considering getting pregnant or have had one or more miscarriages, be sure to let your doctor know of your family history. Women with thrombophilia may be at increased risk for miscarriage, as a blood clot can impair the growth of a developing baby. If thrombophilia runs in your family, or if you have experienced multiple miscarriages, talk to your doctor about assessing your risks and taking any preventive steps that may help.

If you are a woman with a family history of thrombophilia or carry one or more thrombophilia mutations, you may also want to be careful about taking hormonal medications, including birth control pills and hormone replacement therapy. These medicines can increase the risk of blood clots. Talk to your doctor to see if you should avoid these medications.

How You Can Treat Blood Clotting Disorders

If blood clots run in your family, or you have tested positive for thrombophilia mutations, work with your doctor to develop a plan to limit your risk of blood clots. Common preventive steps include:

- Making sure you perform certain exercises during long-distance travel to keep your blood circulating efficiently.
- Losing weight.
- Avoiding cigarettes and other tobacco products.
- Following a regular exercise routine.
- If you're a woman, choosing forms of birth control or menopause treatment that don't rely on additional hormones.
- Taking blood thinners during surgery.

If you've already developed a blood clot, your doctor will likely prescribe blood thinners to break up the clot and keep it from circulating throughout your body. Some people who are prone to blood clots need to take blood thinners on a long-term basis, and undergo regular blood tests to make sure the drugs are working properly.

Blood thinners, however, pose some challenges of their own. Not everyone responds to particular blood thinners in the same way—while the drugs help many people, some find the medicine makes them bleed too easily, while others don't benefit from the medication and remain at risk of blood clots. These potential complications make it essential that a person be given the proper type and dose of blood-thinning drugs.

That balance is being made easier, in some cases, by genomics. Doctors and scientists have determined that many people's response to a commonly prescribed blood thinner, warfarin, rests in their genes. About two million Americans start taking warfarin each year, according to federal health estimates, but about one-third of these patients don't react to the drug as expected. Some of that variability is genetic, and a genetic test can reveal which patients are at greater risk of having unexpected reactions to warfarin. As a result, the prescribing information for warfarin now includes details on relevant genetic tests.

If you and your doctor are considering starting you on warfarin, ask about genetic testing. Your results can help you and your doctor decide if the drug is right for you, or if you should try a different blood thinner.

The Bottom Line on Blood Clotting Disorders

Genes alone can't cause blood clots, but certain mutations can increase your risk. Other genetic variants may determine how you respond to warfarin. If a history of any type of clotting problem runs in your family, talk to your doctor, who can help you decide if genetic tests are right for you or refer you to a specialist for further consultation.

HEMOCHROMATOSIS

Hemochromatosis causes the body to overdose on iron, triggering your cells to absorb and store too much of the iron found in your food. Everyone needs adequate levels of iron for healthy blood, as iron is an essential part of hemoglobin. But if your tissues absorb too much iron, your body has no way to rid itself of the excess. If excess iron winds up in your heart, as well as your liver, pancreas, and other organs, it can build up to toxic levels and cause serious damage. Some people with hemochromatosis develop heart disease or liver cancer as a result of their high iron levels, and some die from the condition. (For the story of one woman's battle with hemochromatosis, see Chapter 1.)

Most cases of hemochromatosis are inherited, although the disease is sometimes acquired after a person receives many blood transfusions, develops long-term liver disease, or takes iron supplements in excessive amounts. Since iron usually takes a long time to reach harmful levels in the body, most of the symptoms and problems associated with hemochromatosis arise later in life, often after the age of 30 in men and 50 in women. Early warning signs include joint pain, fatigue, weakness, and abdominal pain. While juvenile forms of hemochromatosis are much more rare, children occasionally develop the disease.

How Genes Are Involved

Most cases of hemochromatosis arise from mutations in a gene called *HFE* on Chromosome 6. This gene helps regulate iron absorption, and *HFE* mutations can allow too much iron to flow into tissues and organs. Hemochromatosis is inherited in an autosomal recessive manner; a person must inherit two copies of an *HFE* mutation, one from each parent, to develop the disease. Carriers, who have only one copy, face far less risk, but sometimes develop slightly elevated iron levels. *HFE* mutations are among the most common disease-related gene variants found in the United States. The mutations occur most often in Caucasians, especially those of northern European descent. Among this group, about 1 in every 8 to 12 Americans carries one copy of an *HFE* mutation, and about 5 people in every 1,000 carry two copies. Carrier rates are lower for African-Americans, Asian-Americans, Latinos, and other ethnic groups.

An *HFE* mutation, however, is no guarantee of illness. Scientists have learned that even two copies of an *HFE* mutation do not always give rise to hemochromatosis. Some people with the mutations never develop the disease. Scientists are now trying to understand why hemochromatosis affects only some of the people with *HFE* mutations.

Genetic Testing for Hemochromatosis

Tests for the most common disease-related *HFE* mutations, called C282Y and H63D, are now widely available, both through regular doctors and direct-to-consumer genetic testing companies. Doctors usually recommend getting an *HFE* test through an established medical network, which can provide genetic counseling, follow-up testing, and treatment if needed.

If you choose a direct-to-consumer *HFE* test, keep in mind that your test results may not give you the last word on your hemochromatosis status. If your test results are negative, that's great news—your risk for inherited hemochromatosis is very low. If your test results show you are either a C282Y carrier, or have two copies of the mutation, that information alone can't tell you if you have hemochromatosis. People with two copies of the mutation are certainly at increased risk, but since not everyone

---

Hemochromatosis: Not Just a "Celtic" Disease

Hemochromatosis has come to be described as a Celtic disease, reflecting the fact that *HFE* mutations are more common among people of Scottish or Irish origin. In Ireland, for example, as many as 1 in 5 people is a carrier. But carrier rates are also relatively high among other northern Europeans, such as Swedes and Danes. For that reason, health recommendations in the United States say that all people of northern European origin need to be mindful of hemochromatosis.

with an *HFE* mutation gets sick from it, you'll need another test to check levels of iron in your blood. Inherited hemochromatosis also causes health problems over time, so you will need further blood tests to check your iron levels at regular intervals for the rest of your life. If your iron levels are high, you'll need prompt medical attention and will probably be referred to a specialist.

Some people who are concerned about their hemochromatosis risk prefer direct-to-consumer genetic testing to prevent insurance companies from seeing their test results. The relatively low cost of an *HFE* gene test—usually about $200—has boosted the popularity of this form of testing. But think carefully before choosing this route. In case your test results come back positive, make a plan for follow-up care with your doctor. And choose a test from a company that provides genetic counselors who can help you understand and act on your test results.

Special Considerations for Hemochromatosis

Pre-menopausal women with *HFE* mutations carry more protection against hemochromatosis than men, thanks to monthly periods that shed blood—and excess iron—from the body. For this reason, women who develop hemochromatosis from their mutations usually fall ill only after menopause. Men, on the other hand, develop symptoms and hemochromatosis-related illness much earlier, and are about five times more likely to be diagnosed with the effects of hereditary hemochromatosis.

Until the relatively recent discovery of *HFE* mutations and their prevalence, hemochromatosis was considered very rare. While gene experts are very familiar with the condition, not all family doctors recognize the disease or are comfortable with diagnosing hemochromatosis or ordering tests for it. Early symptoms of the disease can be vague, mimicking common conditions that have nothing to do with *HFE* mutations.

Many people with hemochromatosis tell stories of bouncing from doctor to doctor for years before finally being diagnosed. If you are Caucasian and signs of hemochromatosis run in your family—such as men who've had heart attacks at a young age or family members who have developed liver cancer—talk to your doctor about hemochromatosis testing. If your doctor isn't sure about a genetic test for *HFE* mutations, you can start with a more routine, less expensive blood test to check your iron levels. If they are high, a genetic test can then help find the cause and point out the need for other members of your family to be tested, as well.

How You Can Treat Hemochromatosis

Once the disease is diagnosed, treatment is relatively easy, safe, and inexpensive. *HFE* mutations can't be fixed, but excess iron can be removed from your body through periodic blood withdrawal, or phlebotomy. You will be sent to a phlebotomy center that withdraws a pint of blood from your body at each visit, until blood tests show you carry a safe level of iron. The number of withdrawals you'll need depends on how much excess iron you carry.

If your hemochromatosis is caught early, phlebotomy can substantially improve many of the symptoms of the disease and lower your risk of serious illness such as heart disease. If your diagnosis comes later, however, a few of the effects of hemochromatosis, such as joint pain and arthritis, may not show as much improvement. The most dangerous problem arises if excess iron has damaged your liver. If so, you are at increased risk of developing liver cancer, and you'll need regular care from a specialist in liver disease.

The Bottom Line on Hemochromatosis

HFE gene mutations are relatively common among Caucasians, although many people with a mutation don't become ill. If you fit the ethnic profile for hemochromatosis, and symptoms of the illness run in your family, seek a genetic test or blood iron levels test that can help clarify your risks for the disease or diagnose the condition.

IRREGULAR HEARTBEAT

Your heart needs more than strong muscle and a good supply of blood to do its job. It also relies on a steady flow of electricity, which accompanies every heartbeat and keeps your heart pumping in an even rhythm. This voltage is generated within the heart itself, largely by minerals that move through microscopic holes between your heart cells. When you undergo an electrocardiogram, the test traces your heartbeat by measuring this electrical activity.

Most of the time, the heart's electrical system works at a steady pace, keeping your heartbeat strong and even. But when this electrical flow is disrupted, your heart can't continue its reliable rhythm. It may beat erratically, or too quickly, or stop altogether. This irregular heartbeat is called arrhythmia, and it's a very common medical problem. More than two million Americans suffer from some form of arrhythmia. Some cases of irregular heartbeat are mild, requiring little or no treatment. Others require steady doses of medication to even out the heartbeat, or a pacemaker or other electrical device implanted in the chest to restore a regular heartbeat. If a serious arrhythmia hits suddenly, often because a blood vessel that feeds the heart gets blocked, the heart may not be able to keep recharging itself, and could stop altogether without warning. This condition, called sudden cardiac arrest, kills hundreds of thousands of Americans each year, according to the American Heart Association.

Blocked blood vessels aren't the only cause of dangerous irregular heartbeats, however. In some people, faulty genes cause the heart's electrical system to work improperly, especially during times of shock or stress. Here we look at one form of inherited irregular heartbeat called

Reproductive Donors Can Anonymously Notify Potential Biological Offspring of Genetic Information

B randon, his wife, Lisa, and I were reviewing the genetic test results that showed Brandon carried the same Long QT genetic mutation that had caused his brother's premature death. Long QT is a heart condition that results in an abnormal rhythm that can cause a person to faint or, if unchecked, to die. During the session, we discussed testing their children because having this information could help them with lifestyle decisions, such as whether to limit high-intensity sports activities. Brandon looked nervous as we discussed the children, and I assumed he was dealing with some tough emotions. We explored how difficult it is to pass a genetic mutation on to your children because, as parents, we want to do everything possible to protect them. Although you don't have a choice about which genes they inherit, it is emotionally difficult to think that you could have passed a mutated gene on to your child.

But that was only one reason Brandon was anxious when discussing children. He called me a few days later to ask if he could come in for a consultation by himself. And that was when he shared that he had been a regular donor for a sperm bank while in college 15 years ago. Why not? In addition to the money he received for his donations, as a good-looking pre-law student, his were the type of genes that should be shared, right? But now, could there be lots of children who had a 50-percent chance of having the same gene mutation? He had never told Lisa about his sperm donations, and he really didn't want her to know. He didn't want to ever know those kids, but what should he do? He didn't even know if the sperm bank still existed.

With Brandon's permission, I located the sperm bank that had accepted his donations and I helped him draft a letter explaining the new genetic information. He wrote to the sperm bank, but made it clear in the letter that he did not want contact with any potential children. He also gave his cell phone number as his contact because he didn't want his wife to know about that part of his life. A week later, he received a call from the genetic counselor at the sperm bank. She thanked him for the information and told him that they would contact the women who had received vials of his sperm and reported live births. She would assume responsibility to share the information with them. He was also assured that he would not be required to have contact with the children if he didn't want to.

Bottom line: As a genetic counselor, I typically don't ask if men have donated sperm, so I was pleased that Brandon was ethical enough to realize those ramifications of having this mutation. Most accredited sperm banks ask that donors contact them if new medical or genetic information becomes available. The sperm bank will typically assume responsibility for contacting the women who received the specimens and reported success. In this new age of artificial reproductive technologies, donors have even more responsibility to consider the impact of their genetic information on all their biological offspring.

long QT syndrome. While this condition is relatively rare, genomic scientists say that improved understanding of long QT syndrome is helping to unravel the genetics behind more common types of irregular heartbeat.

The syndrome's name refers to part of the natural sequence of a person's heartbeat, called the QT interval. People with long QT syndrome can develop a prolonged interval that leaves their hearts slow to generate the electricity it needs for its next beat. That delay makes their hearts prone to start beating wildly, too quickly and too lightly to pump blood effectively. This dangerous rhythm is called *torsades de pointes*, and when it first strikes, it usually makes a person faint. Sometimes, the heart can correct itself. But if the irregular heartbeat persists, the person will die if their heart isn't shocked back into a normal rhythm.

Once considered extremely rare, long QT syndrome is now believed to be more widespread than previously thought. The syndrome strikes both children and adults, and it is believed to be responsible for some cases of sudden infant death syndrome, as well as many cases of unexplained fainting, cardiac arrest, or drowning death in children and young adults. Exact carrier rates are difficult to determine, as the condition often goes undiagnosed until a person dies unexpectedly of cardiac arrest. For this reason, some experts recommend that people who die from cardiac arrest at a young age undergo an autopsy to help uncover risks their relatives may face. Current scientific estimates say that about every 1 in 5,000 people has some form of inherited long QT, and that about 3,000 Americans die from it each year.

How Genes Are Involved

At least 10 different forms of long QT syndrome have been discovered, each tied to a different gene. All are autosomal dominant, meaning that a person need inherit only one copy of a long QT syndrome gene variant to be at risk for the condition. The most common form, long QT type 1, arises from a gene called *KCNQ1*, located on Chromosome 11. This gene is important to maintaining the heart's electrical balance, and this *KCNQ1* mutation distorts the microscopic holes that allow potassium, an important mineral, to flow as it helps maintain the heart's rhythm. People with long QT type 1 appear to be perfectly healthy until they come under physical stress that throws their heart into an irregular rhythm. Running, swimming, hard chores, or shocking news can all trigger an episode of fainting or cardiac arrest in a person with long QT type 1. This condition caused the deaths of the Roberts brothers, whose story appears at the beginning of this chapter.

Other forms of long QT syndrome involve other elements of the heart's electrical system, and can be triggered by different external forces. People with long QT type 2, for example, can be thrown into a fainting episode or cardiac arrest by surprising noises, including alarm clocks or telephones. In one family that later proved to have long QT type 2, for example, a child died after a relative startled him with a loud "Boo!"

during a game of hide-and-seek. People with long QT type 3, in contrast, often die in their sleep, for reasons scientists are still trying to unravel.

While long QT mutations can be dangerous, they do not always govern how the heart works. For reasons that still aren't clear, some people with a long QT mutation may never develop an irregular heartbeat, faint, or suffer cardiac arrest. Others suffer multiple episodes of fainting or cardiac arrest, or die without any warning at all. A teenage athlete with undiagnosed long QT type 1 may excel during her rigorous swim practices, only to black out when an extra jolt of adrenaline hits during a stressful race. Scientists are working to improve our understanding of how these mutations affect the heart and when they are most likely to harm a person's health.

Genetic Testing for Irregular Heartbeat

A genetic test for five forms of long QT syndrome is now available through doctors' offices. The test is not offered by any direct-to-consumer testing company.

The long QT syndrome genes analyzed by this test explain about 75 percent of all long QT syndrome cases. If your test results are positive, the answers can help shape plans for protecting your own health and point out risks to other family members. But because the test doesn't cover all long QT syndrome genes, a negative test result doesn't mean you are free from all long QT mutations. Also, keep in mind that having a long QT mutation doesn't always mean you'll develop a dangerous irregular heartbeat.

Non-genetic tests, however, are required to conclusively diagnose long QT syndrome. These usually involve a variety of electrocardiograms, some done under physical stress, that reveal the heart's rhythm and any prolonged QT interval. These tests are an essential part of any long QT syndrome diagnosis, and the genetic test is never used as the sole diagnostic tool.

Newer genetic tests are also becoming available for more common types of irregular heartbeat. Genomic scientists hope that studies of syndromes such as long QT will soon reveal more about these conditions and allow more such tests to be developed.

Other Genes, Other Heartbeat Risks

When it comes to irregular heartbeat, scientists are busy looking at more than just long QT syndrome. A genetic variant on Chromosome 1, for example, has been implicated in some cases of atrial fibrillation, a dangerous arrhythmia in the top two chambers of the heart. Given the dangers posed by irregular heartbeat, you can expect to see researchers work on uncovering more genetic factors that increase risk.

Special Considerations for Irregular Heartbeat

Not all cases of long QT syndrome are inherited. More than 50 medications, some of them quite common, can also trigger long QT syndrome. These include certain antibiotics such as Cipro, breathing aids such as Primatene, and antidepressants such as Prozac. The University of Arizona's Center for Education and Research on Therapeutics maintains an up-to-date list of medicines linked to irregular heartbeat at www.arizonacert.org/medical-pros/drug-lists/drug-lists.cfm.

If you experience any heartbeat irregularities or unexplained fainting while taking a medication, let your doctor know immediately, even if you've never had a problem before. Doctors believe some people who otherwise appear healthy may have subtle features in heart-related genes that make them more vulnerable to developing long QT syndrome while taking certain medications. People who know they have inherited long QT syndrome should avoid any drug linked to irregular heartbeat.

How You Can Treat Irregular Heartbeat

Common treatments for more typical cases of irregular heartbeat, including medication and internal devices to control the heart's rhythm, are also used by people with long QT syndrome. Turning to these therapies is rarely an easy choice. Most were developed for the older patients in whom arrhythmias usually occur. Using regular heart medication or an internal heart-starter, or defibrillator, for a small child with long QT syndrome is a difficult decision. It requires frequent follow-up care to make sure the drugs are working properly or subsequent surgeries to replace or repair internal defibrillators. Some specialists recommend against the use of internal defibrillators in young children. Some families still choose them, however, preferring the risks to the possibility of their child dying from cardiac arrest.

If someone near you experiences sudden cardiac arrest from an irregular heartbeat, you have only a few minutes before the person suffers irreversible brain damage or dies. Call 911 immediately, and begin helping the person get air and circulate blood by performing cardiopulmonary resuscitation (CPR). If you don't know CPR, many civic organizations in your community, such as the Red Cross and local hospitals, offer CPR courses for you to take. If an electric defibrillator is nearby, use it to help shock the person's heart back into a normal rhythm. These devices, called automatic external defibrillators, or AEDs, are now commonly found in many public places, including airports, shopping malls, and schools. They are easy to use, require no prior training, and are designed to avoid harming the person they are used on. AEDs have been credited with saving thousands of people, and can literally be a lifesaver until emergency medical help arrives.

The Bottom Line on Irregular Heartbeat

While much remains to be learned about how genes shape your heart's electrical system, research into conditions such as long QT syndrome is paving the way for a more comprehensive genomic approach to arrhythmias. If you have any episodes of unexplained fainting or cardiac arrest in your family history, especially at a young age, talk to a specialist about your own risks for inherited irregular heartbeat. And if you experience any heartbeat problems while taking a particular medication, let your doctor know immediately.

CHOLESTEROL

Cholesterol has become such a culprit in the campaign against heart disease that it's easy to forget that this substance is actually an essential part of your health. This soft, waxy material is found among the fats in your blood and your cells, helping build cell membranes, some hormones, and performing other important jobs. Your body makes some of its own cholesterol, and the rest comes from the food you eat. Only when cholesterol levels in the blood swing too high or too low does cholesterol offer more harm than help.

Two types of cholesterol play a major role in your health—LDL and HDL. LDL, which stands for low-density lipoprotein, is prone to sticking to arterial walls, and is commonly known as bad cholesterol. HDL, or high-density lipoprotein, is known as good cholesterol because it keeps LDL levels under control. A higher level of LDL increases your risk of a heart attack, while a higher level of HDL lowers it.

Many of the little choices you make every day add up to major influences on your cholesterol. If you usually order a cheeseburger for lunch, this high-fat, high-cholesterol meal boosts your own cholesterol levels. A salad, on the other hand, offers vitamin-rich vegetables shown to reduce blood cholesterol. Regular exercise can also drive cholesterol numbers down, while smoking pushes up your health risks by encouraging cholesterol to stick to the walls of your arteries. Americans' high-fat diets and couch-potato lifestyles have helped make high cholesterol a widespread health problem estimated to affect more than 100 million people.

Alongside your choices in food, smoking, and exercise, your genes also play a key role in your cholesterol levels and risk for conditions such as atherosclerosis and coronary artery disease. Several important gene mutations have been identified that affect a person's cholesterol levels, and genomic scientists are rapidly uncovering many others. Another mutation affects how a person responds to cholesterol-lowering medication, a discovery that will help doctors pick the best drugs and doses for people with cholesterol problems.

First we focus on two genes with proven links to cholesterol-related illness—*LDLR* and *APOE*.

How Genes Are Involved

While high cholesterol is a common problem, some families have especially worrisome cholesterol numbers. Cholesterol is measured using a blood test that detects milligrams of cholesterol per deciliter of blood, a measurement expressed in units of mg/dl. For most people, doctors recommend an overall cholesterol level of 200 mg/dl or less, an LDL level of 100 mg/dl or less, and an HDL level of 40 mg/dl or higher. Some families, however, have multiple members with high cholesterol levels—sometimes even 500 mg/dl or higher—that don't drop much even after a change in diet. In these families, some members suffer heart attacks at a relatively young age.

This condition, called familial hypercholesterolemia, is caused by a series of mutations, including one on a gene called *LDLR*. Located on Chromosome 19, this gene carries instructions for an important part of how LDL cholesterol is absorbed by your cells. If someone has a hypercholesterolemia-related mutation on the *LDLR* gene, their cells can't absorb LDL properly, leaving excessive amounts of "bad" cholesterol circulating in the blood. The mutation is autosomal dominant, meaning a person need inherit only one copy to develop very high cholesterol. Men with this mutation are 50 times more likely to have heart attack by the age of 40, and half of them develop coronary heart disease by the age of 60. Women with this mutation are 125 times more likely to have a heart attack by the age of 40, and one-third will develop coronary heart disease by the time they are 60. Along with very high cholesterol levels and increased risk of heart disease and heart attack, people with familial hypercholesterolemia often have fatty deposits on the surface of their skin, a sign that their bodies aren't able to process cholesterol properly.

Familial hypercholesterolemia was once considered rare, but recent research has revealed that this *LDLR* mutation is one of most frequent genetic disorders in the United States. At least 1 in every 500 people—about 600,000 Americans—has a mutation. Among people who've had a heart attack and survived, 1 in every 20 has one copy. Doctors expect that ongoing research will further clarify just how common this *LDLR* mutation really is.

The *APOE* gene comes in three varieties, or alleles, each with its own effects on blood cholesterol levels. The gene, located on Chromosome 19, plays an important role in your body's ability to absorb, process, and remove fats, including cholesterol. Each of the gene's alleles, called *APOE e2*, *APOE e3*, and *APOE e4*, has a different impact on cholesterol and fats in the blood:

- People with two copies of the *APOE e2* allele (about 13 percent of the population) may clear dietary fat from their bodies at a slower rate than normal, and are at somewhat higher risk of early cardiovascular disease. They may also have elevated levels of triglycerides, another type of blood-borne fat linked to heart disease. Two copies of *APOE e2*, however, are no guarantee of heart disease or a heart attack, as many outside factors, including age, diet, and exercise can all enhance or counteract the alleles' effects.

- People with two copies of the *APOE e3* allele (about 62 percent of the population) have the most common form of this gene and have no increased risk of heart disease from this gene. Lifestyle choices, however, may still put them at risk of high cholesterol and heart disease.
- People with two copies of the *APOE e4* allele (about 25 percent of the population) are at increased risk of atheroscelorosis. They may also have elevated levels of trigyclerides. Two copies of *APOE e4*, however, don't guarantee that you'll have heart disease or a heart attack. Many other medical conditions, such as obesity or diabetes, or lifestyle choices such as diet and exercise, may increase or decrease a person's risk.

It's important to keep in mind that *LDLR* and *APOE* don't set your entire cholesterol profile. This is one area in which both a multitude of genes, as well as what you eat, interact to define your health over time. Genomic scientists have already identified hundreds of genes related to cholesterol, and more are constantly coming to light as research uncovers the function of each piece of the human genome. While the medical benefits of these more recently discovered genes aren't yet concrete, scientists are rapidly making new discoveries that help explain why cholesterol concerns vary so much from person to person. Scientists have discovered, for example, that some people with particular gene features develop high cholesterol from a high-fat diet, while others develop it from a diet high in starches and sugars. Over time, these findings will help you better understand your cholesterol risks and follow a diet more likely to keep your cholesterol low and your heart healthy.

Genes also play an important role in how some people respond to cholesterol medication, an element covered a little later in this chapter.

Genetic Testing for Cholesterol Problems

Gene tests for both *LDLR* mutations and *APOE* alleles are available. The *LDLR* test can only be ordered by a doctor, who often pursues it to pinpoint the cause of a patient's very high cholesterol. The test can also be useful for relatives of someone with a confirmed *LDLR* mutation who wants a better sense of their own cholesterol risks.

While most *APOE* tests are also ordered through doctors, a few direct-to-consumer companies sell the test as well. This route to *APOE* testing, however, is extremely controversial, and doctors don't recommend it. This caution stems from the dual role of *APOE*. One variation of *APOE*, *APOE e4*, has also been linked to an increased risk of Alzheimer's disease, making an *APOE* test a complicated medical decision. *APOE e4* and Alzheimer's is discussed more in Chapter 7. If you are interested in an

APOE test for heart disease risk, your most beneficial route is through your doctor.

If you do undergo a genetic test for cholesterol risk, keep in mind that it probably won't answer many of your cholesterol questions. Gene testing isn't the most common or reliable way to diagnose high cholesterol, coronary artery disease, or an imminent heart attack. Both the *LDLR* mutation and *APOE* alleles only increase a person's risk of these problems, rather than directly causing them. And if your test results are negative, you can still develop high cholesterol or coronary artery disease from your diet, lifestyle, and other genes.

The most effective way to diagnose high cholesterol is a simple blood test that measures your levels of overall cholesterol, LDL, HDL, and other fatty substances in the blood. Cholesterol tests are inexpensive, routinely covered by insurance, and easily done through your family doctor. Your family history, along with these cholesterol test results, currently offers you the most valuable insight into your heart health and your risks for heart problems later on. Many doctors also recommend a blood test for a substance called C-reactive protein. The test measures the level of inflammation in your body—an important sign of cardiovascular health.

If your doctor suspects you already have coronary artery disease, or you've survived a heart attack, electronic scans of your heart and coronary blood vessels can further reveal whether you have any risky arterial blockages that need treatment.

Special Considerations for Cholesterol

Given the large number of genes that affect your cholesterol levels and risks for cardiovascular disease, it's no surprise that the causes and effects of high cholesterol vary widely from person to person. Some people eat plenty of beef and eggs and never develop a problem, while others show high LDL numbers even after sticking to a low-fat diet. So far, public health recommendations on controlling cholesterol have been slow to reflect so many different needs and experiences. If you find that standard recommendations don't seem to be a good fit for you—perhaps dietary advice doesn't lower your cholesterol much, or a certain medication doesn't seem to help—take a close look at your family medical history. If possible, draw on the experiences of your relatives to help you and your doctor craft an effective cholesterol-control plan. If your family history doesn't offer much insight, work with your doctor or nutritionist to try different approaches until you find one that brings your cholesterol numbers down.

How You Can Treat Cholesterol Problems

Most efforts to control cholesterol start with a reduced-fat diet and exercise. For some people, these changes are enough to bring their cholesterol numbers down. Others have had more success by following a vegetarian diet extremely low in most forms of fat.

If diet and exercise don't do enough, however, doctors usually recommend statins, a type of cholesterol-lowering drug that can cut cholesterol levels by as much as 40 percent. Currently, doctors often have to resort to some trial and error to determine the right dose of the right statin drug for each patient. Some people respond better to one statin than another, and a few even develop dangerous side effects. But pharmacogenomic research may soon take some of the guesswork out of statins.

Numerous studies have found that different gene features affect how a person responds to a particular statin. Some people with certain gene variations, for example, don't benefit as much from a common statin called Pravachol. Others with a different gene feature are more likely to develop mild to severe muscle problems as a side effect of taking some statins. A relatively small number of people taking statins, for example, develop muscle weakness after starting the drugs. Researchers have linked a majority of those cases to a SNP found on a gene called *SLCO1B1*, found on Chromosome 12. In the future, this type of research will likely lead to

Is a Regular Medical Test Enough?

If high cholesterol runs in your family, genetic testing can help pinpoint the cause. But since these tests can't diagnose high cholesterol itself, some people considering a genetic cholesterol test find themselves wondering if it's really worth it. Can't they rely on regular blood tests to measure their cholesterol?

For patients, this question often stems from concerns about genetic information winding up in medical records, where health insurance companies might see it. Doctors also have concerns, saying that regular non-genetic cholesterol tests offer a very useful, less costly option.

If you aren't sure about a genetic cholesterol test, gene experts say considering the following questions can help you make a decision:

- How likely is it that available tests can find any mutation you may have?
- How important is it to you to find out the cause of your high cholesterol? How important does your doctor think it is?
- If your test results are positive, would you want to share the information with relatives? With your children? If so, how and when?
- How would the privacy of your test results be protected? (For more information on privacy issues, see Chapter 8.)
- Will the test results affect your treatment, or help you make treatment decisions later on?

Your doctor or a genetic counselor can help you sort through answers to these questions. Regular cholesterol blood tests give you a great way to track your cholesterol. While a genetic test might be a good consideration for some families, most people may find that when it comes to cholesterol, genetic testing isn't the "be all, end all."

genetic tests that help doctors prescribe statins more accurately. Cholesterol is also one focus of an emerging genomic treatment that uses a drug to silence a gene that produces high levels of LDL. The medicine works by quashing the gene's ability to release its instructions, stopping the gene's ability to drive up LDL production. The type of science behind the drug is called RNA interference, or RNAi, and while it very new, it is promising enough to have been the focus of a recent Nobel Prize. Chapter 9 looks more closely at RNAi.

If you've already developed severe arteriosclerosis, or the narrowing and hardening of the arteries caused by inflammation and fatty buildup, you'll need treatments more aggressive than statins. Your doctor will probably recommend surgery to open or circumvent blocked blood vessels.

The Bottom Line on Cholesterol

When it comes to this important health issue, everyone really is unique. What drives up cholesterol in one person may lower it in another, and one person's essential medicine may not do another much good. This variety largely stems from genes. But while your DNA is important, plenty of factors under your control play a big role, as well. Your diet, your exercise habits, and your choice to not smoke, can all help lower your cholesterol and keep your arteries clearer, regardless of your genetic tendencies. Awareness of your family history can provide risk information to further reinforce the importance of these healthy lifestyle choices at an early age.

HEART ATTACK

As a life-threatening result of heart disease, heart attacks are understandably feared—and also widely misunderstood. Many people think heart attacks strike suddenly, stopping a person's heart and killing within minutes. But the causes of most heart attacks actually build slowly over long periods of time. And in contrast to the common image of a heart attack victim clutching his chest and falling to the floor, many heart attacks last for hours. Some do serious harm on the inside, but cause such vague symptoms that a person may not realize she is having one.

Heart attacks occur when the heart muscle is starved of the oxygen-carrying blood it needs to keep working. This cutoff usually occurs when one or more of the arteries feeding the heart gets blocked by a buildup of cholesterol deposits—fatty, inflamed plugs that often take decades to develop. Without deliveries of blood and oxygen, heart tissue starts to weaken and die, hurting the heart's ability to do its job. In many people suffering a heart attack, this damage unfolds over a period of hours. While these episodes are often very painful, many people are awake and alert during a heart attack. The dramatic collapses most people associate with heart attacks are actually due to sudden cardiac arrest. While heart attacks sometimes lead to sudden cardiac arrest, this life-threatening heart stoppage actually hits when the heart's rhythm gets out of sync. And as we mentioned earlier in this chapter, such arrhythmia can arise independently of a heart attack.

The fact that many heart attacks unfold gradually, however, doesn't diminish their danger. Every year, about 1.2 million Americans suffer a heart attack, and about 40 percent of them die. Despite improvements in treating heart attacks, preventing these cardiac crises remains a top health concern. Many of the factors that shape your risk of a heart attack—especially your diet, your exercise habits, and your decisions on smoking—are in your control. But genomic scientists are also revealing how genes influence your risk of having a heart attack, or of dying from one if it strikes.

How Genes Are Involved

Scientists have yet to uncover all the genes related to heart attacks, and it's very unlikely that any one gene controls all your heart-attack risk. But a look at several different gene discoveries shows just some of the ways DNA affects different people's chances of having or surviving a heart attack:

- People with one of two variants in a gene called *VAMP8* are about twice as likely to have an early heart attack. *VAMP8* carries the code for a protein important in blood clotting, and if clots form in coronary blood vessels, they can lead to a heart attack.
- Caucasians with a particular variation in a gene called *EPHX2* are about 1-½ times more likely to have a coronary heart disease event such as a heart attack. The gene generates a substance that rids the body of helpful fatty acids, and people with this polymorphism appear to lose these fatty acids too quickly, reducing their protection against heart problems.
- A gene pattern found among some Caucasians and African-Americans in the United States slightly increases the risk of heart attack in whites, but proves much deadlier in blacks. The HapK gene pattern, involving a collection of different polymorphisms, is found more frequently in Caucasians, and increases their risk of heart attack by 16 percent. But African-Americans with the HapK pattern face a much higher risk—as high as 250 percent. HapK appears to affect heart-attack risk by increasing the likelihood that fatty deposits in the arteries will rupture and plug essential blood vessels. Genetic factors such as the HapK pattern are part of the reason why doctors say it is essential that African-Americans receive early preventive care against heart disease.
- The *APOE* gene, described earlier in this chapter's section on cholesterol, also appears to affect survival after a heart attack. One study found that people with *APOE e4* alleles were more likely to die within five years of a heart attack, usually by suffering another heart

attack. But if *APOE e4* heart-attack survivors were treated with cholesterol-lowering statin drugs, that extra risk decreased substantially.

While genomic scientists don't yet have all the answers about genes and heart attacks, the findings they've uncovered so far make it clear that your DNA has plenty to say when it comes to your heart attack risk.

Genetic Testing for Heart Attack Risk

Some direct-to-consumer genetic testing companies now offer analysis of parts of your genome containing SNPs related to heart-attack risk. This analysis is usually part of a larger look at many other disease-related SNPs, and hence is likely to cost at least several hundred dollars. If you choose this type of testing, experts recommend selecting a testing firm that offers a genetic counselor's help in interpreting your test results.

There are also tests available for cholesterol-related genes, which can be a critical part of your risk for a heart attack. These tests are covered in detail in this chapter's section on cholesterol issues.

Special Consideration for Heart Attacks

As the research results just mentioned show, your ethnic background can play a role in your risk of a heart attack. African-Americans, for example, have a higher death rate from heart attacks than whites. Americans from the Indian subcontinent also have a high rate of heart attacks, especially at a young age. Some of the higher risks faced by individual ethnic groups can be explained by external factors such as diet and access to quality medical care. But doctors increasingly believe that genes play a major role. Talk to your doctor about heart-attack risks in your ethnic group, how they affect you, and what you can do to lower your own chances of a heart attack.

IN THE NEWS

For Some, a Heart Attack Could Equal a Gene Plus Java

Doctors have long wondered if coffee consumption somehow boosts the chance of having a heart attack. Now, scientists have discovered that in some people, more coffee each day does increase heart attack risk. In the study of more than 4,000 people—half of whom had suffered a heart attack—researchers found that both coffee and a particular gene played a role. The gene is called *CYP1A2*, and it affects how your body metabolizes caffeine. People in the study with a particular allele of the gene that slows caffeine metabolism had a higher risk of a heart attack if they drank higher amounts of coffee—36 percent higher if they drank two cups of coffee or more per day, and 64 percent higher after four or more cups per day.

You don't need a genetic test, though, to know how much coffee to drink. Scientists say it's a good idea for everyone to avoid drinking more than four cups a day.

How You Can Lower Your Risk of a Heart Attack

While some of your risk may reside in your genes, there are many direct steps you can take to reduce your risk. Here are just a few:

- Understand your family history of heart attacks and heart disease, and discuss that information with your doctor.
- Choose a healthy diet, adding in more fruits, vegetables, and high-fiber foods, and reducing saturated fats and simple carbohydrates.
- Manage your weight, and be especially mindful of excess body fat around the waist. Abdominal fat carries a higher risk of health problems, including heart disease and heart attack.
- Pay attention to signs of high blood sugar, and manage diabetes if you have it. People with diabetes face a much higher risk of heart attack.
- Stop smoking if you do smoke, and avoid exposure to second-hand smoke. Smoking even just a couple of cigarettes a day dramatically increases your risk of heart attack.
- Get regular exercise, aiming for 30 minutes of aerobic exercise three to five times a week.

For more prevention suggestions, talk with your doctor. Your physician can assess your current weight, cholesterol levels, and family history to develop a prevention plan suited to your needs.

The Bottom Line on Heart Attacks

While genes clearly play a role in heart attacks, there are currently few tests available to help clarify your own individual risks. Your family history of heart disease and heart attack, however, can improve your understanding of your risks. And remember that when it comes to heart attacks, prevention is the best medicine. By keeping your cholesterol under control, following a healthy diet, getting regular exercise, and avoiding cigarettes, you can go a long way toward reducing your risk of a heart attack.

FREQUENTLY ASKED QUESTIONS ON GENES AND HEART HEALTH

Q. My family could keep a hospital's cardiac ward in business. Three of my close relatives have had heart attacks, and two have died from them. Many of us have cholesterol levels well over 200. But we all also love fatty food—steaks every Sunday, freezers full of ice cream, and pizza as a regular afternoon snack. How are we supposed to know if we should blame our genes or our diet for our problems?

A. Both your family history and the contents of your refrigerator are likely culprits. You can talk to your doctor about a genetic test for inherited high cholesterol, but your diet would likely skew anyone's cholesterol numbers. If you'd rather not take a genetic test, or your gene test results are negative, you can do yourself and your family a favor by replacing the high-fat foods on your table with more fruits, vegetables, and lean meats and cheese. Your doctor or a nutritionist can help you craft an eating plan better suited to lower cholesterol.

Q. *I've had a couple of unexplained fainting episodes in my life, and my teenage son, a runner, recently blacked out after a track meet. Our family doctor says there are many different causes of fainting, and that we shouldn't worry about having a heart condition, especially a genetic one. I'm still concerned, though, and not sure what to do.*

A. There are indeed many different reasons people faint, and happily, many of them have nothing to do with heart trouble. Some people, for example, become dizzy or faint if their blood sugar falls very low. But any heart specialist who hears your story will tell you that a little additional investigation would be worthwhile. Ask for a referral to a heart specialist, or seek one out yourself. You and your son will probably be given tests that measure your heart's activity and electrical patterns to assess the cause of your fainting.

Q. *I'm about to get married, and my fiancée and I have a true American melting pot story. My parents are from Iran, and my fiancée's family is from Cambodia. We both grew up in Los Angeles, where doctors see lots of people who are immigrants. When I had a recent checkup and told my doctor I was getting married, she mentioned that if we want to have children, we should think about thalassemia carrier testing. But if our families are from such different parts of the world, I don't really see why that's necessary.*

A. Your and your fiancée's different backgrounds definitely give you different genetic heritages—and extra protection against many genetic illnesses. But thalassemia, unfortunately, stems from mutations that affect populations from both Iran and Southeast Asia. Carrier testing involves only a blood test, and millions of expectant parents now undergo it for a variety of conditions, including thalassemia. While your risk of having a child with thalassemia is low, a carrier test can be an easy way to check your risk ahead of time. You can find more information on carrier testing in Chapter 3.

Q. *I have fairly severe atherosclerosis, and would like an* APOE *test to look for a genetic cause, but my doctor is really reluctant to do the test, and advises against it. To me, that's really frustrating. I just want to know if I have a genetic risk for clogged arteries, so that I can tell my kids if they're at risk, too.*

A. Your doctor is probably resisting the test for two big reasons. When it comes to atheroscerosis, the *APOE* test only indicates increased risk, not a definite cause. Your atherosclerosis may be linked to multiple genetic variants that the *APOE* test doesn't pick up, so the test likely won't answer your question regarding the cause. Furthermore, one *APOE* allele—*APOE e4*—is also linked to a somewhat increased risk of Alzheimer's disease. Many people don't want to know if they have this risk, as the test can't tell them if they definitely will or won't get Alzheimer's, and there is little they can do to prevent the disease anyway. Before you pursue *APOE* testing further, ask your doctor for a referral to a genetic counselor. You have a lot to consider before deciding that this test is right for you. You'll find more information on the *APOE* test and Alzheimer's disease in Chapter 6.

Q. *A few years ago, to avoid a heart attack, I had to just pay attention to my cholesterol. Now I have to pay attention to types of cholesterol, plus think about blood clots, and worry about inflammation! How am I supposed to keep track of so many things I can't even see, let alone think about how my genes affect everything?*

A. It's true that keeping your heart healthy looks more complicated than it used to be. But the confusion stems more from the way the practice of medicine has traditionally divided things up than any new physical twists. For hundreds of years, medicine has looked at the body in terms of its big physical components—the heart, the lungs, or the colon, for example. But a better understanding of human biology, including human genes, has shown how all these systems are truly intertwined.

Still, tracking your heart health doesn't have to be too complicated. Many of the complex internal processes that affect heart disease—your cholesterol levels, your level of inflammation, sometimes even relevant genes—can be revealed through simple blood tests. Your doctor can help you track your numbers, and over time, help you peer into more and more of your genes. It's definitely more information to keep track of, but the benefits to your health are well worth it.

KEEP IN MIND

If you want to turn to your genes to boost your heart health, these key points can help you make the most of your DNA.

When you are working to keep your heart healthy, you've got a lot more than just your heart to think about. Your blood, your blood vessels, your body's level of inflammation, and even your blood sugar all play a role in cardiovascular health.

Given how many parts of your body affect your heart health, it's no surprise that thousands of genes get involved, as well. Some of these genes are still being researched, but scientists have already made important discoveries that give you and your doctors new tools to track your risks of blood-related illness, high cholesterol, and heart disease.

While your ethnic background plays a big role in all aspects of your health, it's especially important when it comes to heart disease. Talk to your doctor about special risks you may face because of your ethnic background, even if you are young and healthy. The information can let you start taking important preventive steps now.

Gene tests for some cardiovascular conditions may not yet be available, but that doesn't stop you from having at least some understanding of how your genes affect your heart. Together with blood tests for cholesterol and C-reactive protein, a thorough family medical history that includes heart health information offers valuable clues.

And remember that while your cardiovascular genes have plenty of say, so do you. You can override the effects of some harmful gene features and lower your heart-disease risk by following a healthy diet, reducing stress, getting exercise, and avoiding cigarettes. When it comes to your heart, your choices often have more influence than your genes.

Making those choices, though, draws on a part of your body higher than your heart—the gray matter between your ears. Chapter 7 looks at your brain, and how genes get involved in your actions, thoughts, and personality.

CHAPTER SEVEN

YOUR GENES, YOUR BRAIN AND YOUR MENTAL HEALTH

Kendra and Kamika Blake shared their own special language. As little girls, the identical twins made up words only they could understand, making each other laugh when their conversation stumped their parents at the dinner table. Both gifted musicians like their father, the girls learned to play beautiful piano duets. When they weren't at the keyboard, they could often be found inside a playhouse built just big enough for the two of them, sharing books or making up stories about their favorite matched pair of dolls.

As sisters with the same birthday and the same set of genes, Kendra and Kamika loved the way life had made them best friends from the very beginning. As they entered their teen years, though, a sudden shift in their family raised questions about whether their shared genetic heritage might hide a challenge amid all its many gifts.

The girls' mother, Brenda, developed debilitating depression after the death of a beloved aunt who had helped raise her. Brenda's exhausting bouts of bleak sadness made her withdraw from her family for weeks, spending most of the day in bed. The daughters, worried about their mother, wondered what her illness would mean for their family. Kamika, always a little more reserved than her sister, withdrew into the family home as well, handling the cooking and cleaning as she tried to fill her mother's shoes. For Kendra, however, the atmosphere at home made her want to fly out the front door. A friend at school had joined the tennis team, and urged Kendra to try out. With a little coaching, Kendra sharpened her skills on the court enough to take refuge in the sport. When tennis season ended, she took up long-distance running. The greater her worries were at home, the more she played and practiced.

Slowly, with the help of a trusted therapist and antidepressant medication, Brenda overcame her depression. But every improvement she made seemed to be matched by a slide in Kamika's state of mind. Setbacks in high school and college—a poor grade in physics, an insensitive boyfriend, or a botched job interview—sent Kamika into deep depressions of her own. Kendra, on the other hand, stuck to sports as a trusted boost to her own emotional balance. She started trying to help her sister in the same way, taking Kamika on long walks, during which the two sisters could talk and find comfort in their tight connection.

The way these twins share—and don't share—some of the traits most essential to their personalities reflects one of the most fascinating aspects of genomic science and personalized medicine. Just as with any other part of our bodies, our genes shape our brains, carrying the code for everything from basic survival functions to the sophisticated nuances that drive our thoughts, feelings, and creativity. Your genes are an important part of the health of your nervous system, but they're also a key DNA of your personality and mental health. In this chapter we look at how your genes affect everything from basic brain health and development to moods and mental balance. We also cover other influences that shape these aspects of your health, and how you can put them to work with your genes to boost your well-being.

YOUR GENES AND YOUR BRAIN

Did You Know **?**

The next time you have something to say, you are getting help from *FOXP2*, a gene closely tied to human beings' unique ability to speak. This gene, found on Chromosome 7, is a multi-tasker, shaping the way many other genes do their job. While other creatures also carry this gene, the human form of *FOXP2* appears to enable key brain and physical developments that make speech and language possible. Scientists are now working to pinpoint all the ways this gene enables this uniquely human skill. Along the way, they hope studies of *FOXP2* will shed light on many more genes that shape human behavior and character.

When it comes to our thoughts and personality, we human beings like to think of ourselves as creatures of habit and choice. But genomic studies of our brains and personalities reveal that when it comes to our mental health and behavior, we are also creatures of our DNA. The brain, our body's control center, is built and operated by genes.

Some of your genes, for example, carry the instructions for the more primitive parts of your brain. Without any conscious effort on your part, these areas control your heartbeat, breathing, and body temperature—all functions essential for life. They also shape some of your basic emotional responses. Anger, aggression, sadness, and fear all stem from less sophisticated areas of your brain. Other genes shape the more advanced sections of your brain, which control features such as your mood, your intelligence, your memories, complex emotions, and even your creativity.

Your brain handles all these complex tasks with the help of a special communication system that keeps your brain cells working together—and the genes that shape this system are a great example of just how influential these pieces of your DNA can be. Communication between brain cells happens because of neurotransmitters, special chemicals that act as messengers from one nerve cell to another. Your body makes many different neurotransmitters, building them and helping them flow using instructions carried in your genes.

Important Lessons from Genetic Pioneers

Our improving understanding of how genes affect the human brain and our neurological health comes, in part, from the brave work of a group of people who started confronting genetic issues long before most of us.

These people have Huntington's disease, a fatal, inherited condition that usually appears in middle age and slowly destroys brain cells. Caused by a string of bases that repeat themselves too often in a gene on Chromosome 4, Huntington's disease destroys a person's ability to think, feel, and move normally. The illness is especially cruel in its relative ease of discovery but impossibility of recovery—doctors can diagnose Huntington's disease, but can do nothing to stop it. A parent with Huntington's disease has a 50 percent chance of passing the mutation on to each child, making the disease a daunting prospect for entire generations of affected families.

But these grim facts have left people with Huntington's disease, along with their doctors, anything but helpless. Although it is rare, striking about 1 in 10,000 people, Huntington's disease is a giant in the world of genomic medicine. Doctors realized the familial nature of the disease early on, and launched an intense search for the Huntington mutation in the 1980s. That work paid off in 1993, making a genetic test for Huntington's disease possible. That test improved diagnosis of the condition, but also left families with Huntington's disease to grapple with some complex issues in genomic care. How exactly does the Huntington mutation cause damage in the brain? When might symptoms appear? Do people with symptoms of the disease want a genetic test? Do their relatives or their children want a test before they fall ill? Do they want to join medical or genetic experiments? How do insurance companies treat people with the mutation?

Each Huntington's family has its own answers to these questions. But as pioneers in the new world of blending genes and health, some people affected by Huntington's disease actively share their experiences, hoping the lessons they've learned can help us all. Scientists are working on genomic research that might ease or cure Huntington's disease. It's the least they can do, they say, for a group of people who have bravely helped open new genomic doors for everyone.

One of these neurotransmitters, a substance called serotonin, helps your brain regulate your mood, sleep habits, and appetite. Dozens of genes appear to build or influence this neurotransmitter. One important one, the *5-HTT* gene, affects how serotonin travels between your brain cells. If serotonin is flowing in your brain effectively, the aspects of your life affected by serotonin—your mood, your sleep, and your appetite—have a better chance of proceeding normally. But if serotonin doesn't flow normally, or your body's level of serotonin falls too low, these functions might get thrown off balance. You might find your sleeping or eating disrupted, or your mood depressed. Serotonin is known to play an important role in depression, a common mental health issue we look at more closely later in this chapter.

Studies of identical twins like Kendra and Kamika, for example, offer more insights into how genes shape our brain function. As two people who share the same DNA, identical twins often have plenty of mental and personality features in common. Many identical twins share similar talents or special abilities, such as a good eye for drawing or a knack for acing chemistry tests. They also tend to share many aspects of their mental health. If one identical twin generally describes himself as a happy person, studies have found there's a good chance the other will, as well. Identical twins are also more likely to share mental health problems. If one twin suffers from alcoholism or the developmental disorder autism, for example, scientists have discovered that there is a greater chance the other twin will too.

Discovering the Genetics of Addiction

Serotonin isn't the only neurotransmitter undergoing investigation by genetic experts. Another important chemical in your brain, called dopamine, is linked to feelings of pleasure and desire, such as those some people get from alcohol or cigarettes. Dopamine's flow in your brain is partly controlled by a gene called *DRD2*. A few scientific studies have found that people with addictions, such as alcoholics or smokers, tend to have a certain allele of this gene. So far, those insights haven't translated widely into genetic tests for addiction. But scientists hope that ongoing understanding of the genetics of addiction will one day make it easier for some people to reduce their dependence on potentially harmful habits such as smoking or drinking.

YOUR GENES AND YOUR MIND

These discoveries about genes, the brain, and personality fall into a category of genomic science called behavioral genetics. While this is one of the most interesting areas of gene sciences, it's also one of the most controversial. Most people are deeply uncomfortable with the idea that the whole of human identity—including our reason, values, and dreams—can be explained by genes, chemicals, and brain function. What about that part of us that aspires to something higher? How much of us is shaped by that ephemeral force we call the mind or the human spirit, and how much simply comes down to the chemical instructions carried in our genes? What about human creativity, emotions like empathy, and our ability to love? Do these add up to nothing more than bits of DNA code?

These questions also apply to how we act. If behavior is spelled out in the genes, what does that say about a person's responsibility for their own actions? Do our genes mean we really don't have much power to choose what we believe or how we feel? Genes may build the brain, say critics of behavioral genetics, but it's a big leap to go from explaining brain function to defining the human psyche, will, and spirit.

The "Smart Gene"

A few years ago, scientists made big headlines by announcing they had discovered genes that boost the power to learn and remember, and help keep the brain young. Dubbed smart genes, these bits of DNA raised talk of new treatments that could give us all a few more IQ points.

A closer look at the science behind smart genes, however, makes it clear that any everyday benefits from these discoveries are a long way off. To begin with, these findings came from experiments in mice, and the leap from making an Einstein mouse to making a smarter person is a big one. These genes also represent a small fraction of the DNA involved in shaping your memory and intelligence. In addition, the scientists behind these studies made it clear they weren't interested in using their findings to develop some kind of smart pill. Instead, they'd prefer to see understanding of these genes eventually used to help people with neurological problems such as Alzheimer's disease or Down syndrome.

So if you'd like a stronger memory or a higher IQ, you're better off sticking to tried and true brain boosters. Other studies have shown that even small regular bursts of mental activity—doing math by hand instead of reaching for a calculator, or entertaining yourself with a brain-teasing puzzle instead of a night of TV—do a lot to flex the gray matter between your ears.

Gene experts, however, usually don't share these misgivings. Their work shows, time and again, that the genes linked to the brain are just like any other genes at work in our bodies. They hold a great deal of power. But they don't have the last word on how our brains function, what we think, or how we feel. The identical-twin studies that showed a strong role for genes in behavior and mental health have also found that these genes have limits. While identical twins have an increased chance of sharing a particular talent or psychological trait, they don't share these features 100 percent of the time. Not all identical twins develop matching cases of depression or autism.

As with Kendra and Kamika, other influences in our lives also have a powerful effect on our personalities and behavior. Most kids, regardless of their genetic tendencies, spin into a burst of distracted hyperactivity after a sugary treat. For most of us, a bad bout of the flu drains mental and physical energy. A stroll on a sunny day, on the other hand, can help many people lift a blue mood. And habits, especially those passed on through our families, have especially strong influence. In Kendra and Kamika's family, is Kamika's depression caused by a gene inherited from her mother, or by a lifetime of subtle lessons learned from watching her mother cope with difficulty? This question crops up frequently in discussions of behavioral genetics. Addictions, such as alcoholism, often seem to run in families. Scientists have even found a few genes that might be linked to an increased risk of alcoholism or other addictions. But there's no general agreement on whether the children of alcoholics tend to wind up drinking heavily themselves because of genes inherited from their parents or habits copied from them.

In the end, most behavioral geneticists say that both genes and outside influences are critical to our brains, personalities, and mental health. That dual answer might seem vague or frustrating. But it also offers plenty of hope to people worried about inheriting a mental health problem, and puts many important issues affecting your mental well being in your hands. While your genes are a key part of your personality and mental health, they aren't the last word. Your surroundings and your choices are a key part of shaping who you are and how you feel.

To get a more detailed picture of how this dance between genes and other factors shapes your brain, development, and mental health, here is a look at five conditions in which the role of genes is clearly understood. The genes behind these common health concerns not only affect your risk for these conditions, but also offer the promise that our treatments for these challenges will only continue to improve.

DEPRESSION

Once thought to amount to little more than a big dose of blue mood, depression is now recognized as a serious disorder that affects physical well being along with a person's behavior, thoughts, and attitude. Severe depression affects all aspects of a person's life. The condition often brings debilitating physical effects, such as deep fatigue or loss of appetite. It also carries painful mental symptoms such as persistent sadness, anxiety, and a loss of enjoyment in life. The most serious forms of depression can leave people feeling hopeless, sometimes even contemplating suicide. While we all face rough patches in our lives, depression is far more serious, making it difficult for many people to go about their lives for long periods of time.

The condition affects about 17 million Americans of all ages and ethnic backgrounds, according to medical estimates. But the commonplace nature of depression doesn't make the illness any easier to understand. Some people with depression may only suffer one or two bouts of the illness in their lives. For others, depression is a chronic problem. In some, the triggers for depression are clear—the death of a loved one, a painful breakup, or serious financial problems. In others, though, depression seems to arise on its own, with no clear external cause.

Depression comes in several major forms:

- **Major depression** is marked by a deeply sad, hopeless mood that lasts for more than two weeks and comes with some of the physical signs of serious depression, such as major changes in eating, sleeping, or the ability to concentrate.
- **Post-partum depression** hits many women after childbirth, draining them of emotional and physical energy and often leaving them struggling with the responsibilities of being a parent.
- **Seasonal affective disorder** is a pattern of depression that ebbs and

flows with changes in the seasons, especially the approach of winter in cold-weather climates.

- **Bipolar disorder,** once commonly called manic-depressive disorder, is marked by mood swings that sway between emotional highs and deep depression.
- **Dysthymia** is a chronic, low-grade form of depression that is less serious than major depression.
- **Adjustment disorders with depressed mood** encompass emotional symptoms of depression that follow a stressful event, such as death or divorce.
- **Depression with psychosis** is a rare but serious illness in which the emotional and physical symptoms of depression are joined by delusions or hallucinations.

The one clear foundation underlying all these forms of depression is a change in the brain's chemistry. People with depression experience changes in the flow of essential chemicals that affect mood, including serotonin, the neurotransmitter described earlier in this chapter.

How Genes Are Involved

Our bodies don't carry one single depression-related gene. Instead, a mix of different genes appears to contribute to a person's risk of depression. Genes also affect how a person's body responds to antidepressant medication. While many of these genes remain under study, a few have been clearly identified and now factor into some treatment decisions for depression.

One of these key genetic factors is a family of genes called CYP450, found on Chromosome 4. These genes play an important role in how your body processes foreign substances, including medications such as those used to treat depression.

Another key gene is *5-HTT*, found on Chromosome 17. This gene affects how serotonin flows in the brain. This gene's function is shaped by a section of DNA nearby called 5-HTTLPR, which comes in two variations. One of these alleles has been linked to a higher risk of depression after a stressful experience. In one gene study of a group of people in their 20s, for example, 33 percent of those with a risk-related version of the 5-HTTLPR allele developed depression after enduring four or more stressful events, compared with 17 percent of those with another version.

Scientists have also linked this allele to a person's response to some medications used to treat depression. People with the allele that makes them more prone to depression also appear to benefit less from a common group of antidepressant drugs called selective serotonin reuptake inhibitors, or SSRIs. Common antidepressants such as Prozac, Zoloft, and Paxil are all SSRIs. Instead, some doctors say, compounds that don't affect serotonin in the same way may be more effective in people with this allele.

Genetic Testing for Depression

There is no single gene test that can tell you whether you are at risk for depression or if any bouts of depression you have suffered are genetically linked. Depression is a complex condition, and it is likely that many different genes and SNPs affect risk. Any family history of depression, however, is worth noting. If others in your family suffer from depression, you may be at higher risk for developing the condition.

Insights into the CYP450 and 5-HTTLPR genes, however, can sometimes improve your treatment options. If you suffer from depression and choose to take prescription antidepressants, tests that reveal which versions of these genes you carry may help your doctor decide which antidepressant might work best for you. These drugs often work differently from person to person and sometimes cause unpleasant side effects such as dry mouth, blurred vision, nausea, agitation, and sleep disruption. Some people find these side effects so disruptive that they switch to a different antidepressant or drop the medications all together.

The CYP450 test can help reveal whether a person's body is likely to process particular antidepressants effectively. The 5-HTTLPR test can reveal whether a person is likely to respond well to SSRIs or if other drugs

RED FLAG!

Genetic Tests for Mental Conditions: Special Cautions

The uncertainties that limit the usefulness of an HTTLPR test for depression risk also apply to other genetic tests for brain and mental disorders. While the role of genes is clear in a few neurological conditions, such as familial Alzheimer's disease, the influence of genes isn't as well understood in many other problems.

If you are considering any genetic test related to your brain or mental health, especially a direct-to-consumer test, here are some questions to ask up front:

- What exactly does this test look for? Have the genes the test analyzes been conclusively linked to a particular condition?
- Do the genes being tested cause a disease? Or do they point out increased risk? Remember, greater risk is not the same thing as a guarantee of becoming ill.
- Will the test provide any information that affects your medical treatment or health plans? Can you use the information to keep yourself healthier, or does the test point to risks you can't do anything about?
- How often is the test used by other people with your condition, or others who are at risk for the condition you're curious about?

Even if you choose a genetic test through a direct-to-consumer company, consider discussing these issues with your doctor or a genetic counselor beforehand. The answers to these questions can help you make sure you're taking a test that provides information you'll find valuable.

should be prescribed first. These genetic tests must be ordered through your doctor.

Some doctors have welcomed these tests as a way to take some of the guesswork out of prescribing antidepressants. But many also point out their limitations. These tests can only show if certain medications are unlikely to help your depression. While that can be valuable information, it doesn't say which drugs will work, meaning you may still have to try more than one to find the right fit. The tests also only gauge a person's response to certain types of antidepressants, and they don't cover every type of antidepressant.

Special Considerations for Depression

If you are interested in a genetic test to gauge your body's response to particular antidepressants, you may have to pay the costs—often $500 or $600 per test—yourself. Many insurance companies cover antidepressant medications. But some are only willing to pay for these gene tests if a person has unsuccessfully tried several different antidepressants. Some consider the tests too new, and won't pay for them at all. Talk to your insurance company about their policy on paying for CYP450 or 5-HTTLPR testing before deciding on these tests.

How You Can Treat Depression

Millions of Americans rely on antidepressants to keep their depression under control and live happy, fulfilling lives. It's important to note, though, that the growing use of these drugs is controversial, especially in children and teenagers and among adults with milder forms of depression. Critics say that these drugs may be dangerous for some children and teenagers with depression, actually increasing their risk of suicide in some cases. Federal rules now require that antidepressants carry stronger warning labels spelling out the risks to younger people. Some adults with milder forms of depression find that other treatments, such as talk therapy, regular exercise, and plenty of emotional support from family and friends, are enough to lift their depression and let them return to their normal lives. If you have depression, you don't need to suffer alone. Talk to your doctor about all your treatment options to choose an approach that reflects the severity of your depression, your comfort with taking medication for long stretches of time, and how you'd best like to care for your mental health over the long term.

ALZHEIMER'S DISEASE

Fewer diseases of aging raise more concern for most of us than Alzheimer's disease, a progressive illness that steals memory and skills for daily living as it slowly, irreversibly damages the brain. The most common form of dementia, Alzheimer's disease usually strikes people over the

Make Sure You Are Fully Informed When Making Decisions in Complex Genetic Situations

D ave knew that he had cholesterol problems, but he didn't have time to be sick. He traveled a lot, and being on the road with irregular hours and business meetings was not conducive to regular exercise and healthy meals. During an annual check-up mandated by his company for all executives, his doctor once again warned Dave to get his weight and his cholesterol under control. This year, she also drew blood for several tests, including an *APOE* analysis to help determine whether he needed to go on medication and, if so, what type might be best for him. Dave had never heard of *APOE* , but he was glad the test results suggested that he take medicine, because a daily pill would be much easier than trying to find the gym in every hotel and watch his diet.

A couple of years later, Dave's life took on a new crisis. He could no longer ignore the signs that his mother, who he absolutely adored, was developing Alzheimer's disease. After one more major business conference he was going to have to change his position in the company to stay in town, since he was the only one available to care for her. His mom suggested that she spend days in an assisted care facility so he would not worry while he was at work. Her best friend recently moved there, and though she would have preferred being at home, she did not want to be a burden to her son. As part of the intake process, she underwent a number of tests, one of which vaguely sounded familiar. His mother's *APOE* phenotype supported her diagnosis of Alzheimer's disease.

APOE—wasn't that the test his doctor had ordered for his cholesterol problem? Dave asked his mother's doctor about the test. Are there other reasons, like high cholesterol, that someone would have that test? The more he learned, the more nervous Dave became. His cholesterol was now well controlled with medication, but could the test he had taken also provide information about his own chances of someday developing Alzheimer's disease? And why wasn't he told this when he took the test in the first place? What if the information became available to his employer? He was asking for a huge promotion to stay in town, and if the company thought he couldn't handle the job...

Dave called me to ask about the *APOE* test and how he should handle it. It had not raised any flags for the company several years ago, and Dave was busy dealing with his mother's health status. He really didn't want to know if the *APOE* was suggestive of an increased risk for Alzheimer's. Therefore, I suggested he write a letter to his doctor to ensure that information would not be inadvertently disclosed to him.

Bottom line: As a genetic counselor, I spend a lot of time helping patients make fully informed decisions. But it has to be a partnership—we provide the information, and the patients learn and use the information to make decisions that work best for them. In the busy and complicated world of medicine, it is too easy to assume that the health care provider knows what is best for you and to just "do what the doctor says." I encourage you to ask questions and know the consequences of what is happening, even if it is just "a simple blood test."

age of 65. While a little forgetfulness is a common part of aging, the memory loss caused by Alzheimer's disease is far more devastating, often leaving people unable to recall or recognize the most familiar aspects of their lives. Alzheimer's disease often destroys other essential mental capabilities as well, including the abilities to reason, learn, communicate, and make decisions. Over time, many people with Alzheimer's disease lose their capacity to handle simple daily tasks such as getting dressed, making a meal, or running errands. They often stop recognizing relatives or close friends, and may develop personality traits or behaviors that they didn't show before, such as anxiety or suspicion. Eventually, Alzheimer's disease can kill by harming parts of the brain essential to sustaining life. There are currently no major preventive treatments or cures, although a few prescription medications can ease symptoms of the condition for a relatively short period of time.

The graying of the U.S. population makes Alzheimer's disease an increasingly pressing health problem. More than five million Americans have the condition—more than double the number seen in 1980—according to federal health figures. In less than 50 years, that number could reach 16 million.

Age is the single greatest risk factor for Alzheimer's disease. About 1 in every 10 people older than 65 have the condition, and that figure leaps to 1 in 2 among people over 85. Along with age, scientists believe that factors outside a person's brain, such as their overall cardiovascular health, play a role in the development of Alzheimer's disease. People with high blood pressure, diabetes, and high cholesterol, for example, are at greater risk of Alzheimer's disease. But emerging genomic science has also revealed that genes play a direct role in some cases of the disease, and probably increase the risk of the disease in many more people.

How Genes Are Involved

The most direct links between genes and Alzheimer's disease have been found so far in families with members who develop the condition at a much younger age than normal—sometimes as young as their 30s or 40s. These cases of inherited, or familial, early onset Alzheimer's disease are rare, but the mutations seen in these families offer valuable insights into how genes affect the condition. Families with this type of early onset Alzheimer's disease show mutations in one of three genes— *PSEN1*, found on Chromosome 14; *PSEN2*, found on Chromosome 1; and *APP*, found on Chromosome 21. These genes all appear to affect production of amyloid beta, a sticky piece of protein that can form clumps in the brain. The collection of these clumps, or plaques, is linked to the death of brain cells—a process considered significant in the development of Alzheimer's disease.

People with an Alzheimer's-related mutation on one of these genes are almost certain to develop the condition, often in middle age. They also have a 50 percent chance of passing the mutation on to a child.

Most cases of Alzheimer's, however, follow a different pattern, showing less direct family inheritance and appearing later in life. Other genes have been linked to this more common, later-onset form of Alzheimer's disease. These genes, while significant, carry a lower level of risk than the genes related to early-onset Alzheimer's disease. The best known of these late-onset genetic factors is the *APOE* gene, found on Chromosome 19. This gene carries the instructions for making a protein that carries cholesterol in your blood, and comes in several alleles. The most common of these are *APOE e2*, *APOE e3*, and *APOE e4*. (For more information on *APOE*'s role in cholesterol, see Chapter 6.)

Two of these alleles have been linked to Alzheimer's disease risk. While *APOE e3*, the most common form of this gene, doesn't appear to affect Alzheimer's risk, *APOE e2* seems to offer some protection against the disease. *APOE e4*, however, appears to increase the risk of developing Alzheimer's disease. Scientists have found that up to 50 percent of people who develop later-onset Alzheimer's disease have at least one copy of the *APOE e4* allele. Studies have shown that those who have two copies of *APOE e4* are at even greater risk than those with just one copy. While scientists aren't yet sure how these alleles contribute to Alzheimer's disease risk, some think these alleles could affect the flow of cleansing blood through your brain. Others suspect the *APOE* gene may affect your body's ability to clear away tiny clumps of amyloid-beta.

A SNP in a more recently-discovered gene, *CALHM1*, has also been linked to increased risk for late-onset Alzheimer's disease. This gene, found on Chromosome 10, helps shape the flow of calcium in your brain. Scientists hope the gene's discovery will improve our understanding of how Alzheimer's disease develops, perhaps eventually pointing the way to better prevention or treatment.

Genetic Testing for Alzheimer's Disease

Doctors routinely offer genetic tests to families with cases of early onset Alzheimer's disease or confirmed familial Alzheimer's mutations. Family members already showing signs of the illness are often tested to confirm an Alzheimer's diagnosis, while others who are healthy may choose to be tested as well to see if they carry a disease-linked mutation. People with a familial Alzheimer's mutation also often opt for some form of embryonic or pre-natal genetic testing while pregnant or planning a family. Occasionally, however, some people from families with known early onset Alzheimer's mutations decide against testing, because they'd rather not know about impending illness that they can do little to stop.

Gene tests for *APOE* alleles to assess Alzheimer's risk are also available, either through Web-based genetic testing companies or some physicians. The companies that offer *APOE* analysis say that *APOE* information is an important part of long-term health planning. Some doctors may also test for *APOE e4* to help confirm an Alzheimer's disease diagnosis in a person who already shows signs of the illness.

When Families Don't Agree on Genetic Tests

Genes may run in the family, but choices about them sometimes don't. Some members of a family may want to know about genetic risks in detail. Others don't. They find the information too frightening, or believe that a negative test result will cast a shadow over their lives.

These worries are especially common in genetic testing for gradual neurological disorders that can't be prevented or cured, such as familial Alzheimer's disease or Huntington's disease (see more information on Huntington's disease on page 173). Genetic counselors sometimes see complicated family situations such as a father at risk of Huntington's disease who doesn't want to be tested, but a son who does. Since the son's test result could reveal whether the father carries the gene for Huntington's disease, the son's testing decision will ripple throughout the family.

If you are contemplating genetic testing, especially testing for conditions such as familial Alzheimer's disease, here are some questions that can clarify the decision for you and your family:

- Which of your relatives could be affected by your test results?
- How does each of these relatives feel about testing? Do they want to know if they carry a risk-related gene? Or would they rather not know what might lie ahead?
- What are the reasons behind each family member's views on testing? It's harder to reach agreement on genetic tests if everyone's views aren't clear.
- How will your family handle test results that aren't shared? Will the topic be off-limits entirely? What if relatives who don't want to know change their minds later? Decide ahead of time how these situations will be handled.
- Will the test results affect your medical care or plans for staying healthy? If so, will any of these changes inadvertently reveal your test results to your relatives?
- How do you feel about knowing information that you can't share? Will you be comfortable withholding a genetic test result that could affect a close relative too?

These testing situations are understandably complicated. In making your decision, seek the input of a genetic counselor who specializes in neurological conditions. Chances are good he or she has encountered a similar situation before and has helpful insights for how the whole family can face this decision.

It is important to note, however, that many genetic experts and Alzheimer's specialists don't recommend *APOE* testing as a way to for most people to gauge their own Alzheimer's risk. That caution reflects the uncertainty of *APOE* results, along with the limited ability medicine currently has to prevent Alzheimer's in people with higher risk. While *APOE e4* is linked to increased Alzheimer's risk, many people with one or two *APOE e4* alleles never develop Alzheimer's disease. Many others who do develop Alzheimer's don't carry an *APOE e4* allele. Many experts say

APOE results may only cause needless worry for some people, and create a false sense of security for others.

Commercial genetic tests for other genetic factors related to Alzheimer's risk, such as *CALHM1*, will likely become available as these genes and SNPs are better understood. Until doctors have better Alzheimer's preventions and treatments, however, experts usually caution against the widespread use of these tests, as well.

Special Considerations for Alzheimer's Disease

While Alzheimer's disease appears frequently in older people of all racial backgrounds, African-Americans may face higher risks. According to the Alzheimer's Association, a leading support and advocacy group for people with the disease, Alzheimer's disease is anywhere from 14 to 100 percent more prevalent among African-Americans than Caucasians. The reasons for this difference remain unclear. They may lie in genes. The larger number of cases among African-Americans may also reflect the way that poor cardiovascular health appears to increase Alzheimer's disease risk. African-Americans tend to suffer from cardiovascular illnesses, such as high blood pressure, more often.

How You Can Treat Alzheimer's Disease

There is no cure for Alzheimer's disease, and current treatments offer only limited help. A few commercially available medications sometimes ease symptoms of the disease, but any benefits from these drugs are limited and usually fade over time. Hundreds of research efforts to find better preventions and treatments are underway, and scientists hope they will yield promising results over the next decade.

Doctors say your best approach to Alzheimer's disease lies in keeping yourself healthy early in life, long before your risks for the disease rise. Scientists increasingly say that a healthy flow of blood through the brain can reduce Alzheimer's disease risks. When you take steps to reduce your chances of heart disease or stroke, you may also be cutting your risk of Alzheimer's. (For more information on high cholesterol and other cardiovascular conditions, see Chapter 7.) Reducing your risks of diabetes, or keeping your diabetes under control if you already have the condition, may also lower your Alzheimer's risk, as higher blood sugar levels are linked to higher rates of cardiovascular illness.

AUTISM AND PERVASIVE DEVELOPMENT DISORDERS

Autism, a complex neurological condition, has pushed its way to the forefront of childhood health concerns. About one in every 150 children in the United States eventually develops some form of autism, and the condition affects more than one million Americans. As one of the fastest-growing developmental disorders in developed countries, autism consumes the attention of many researchers, doctors, and educational therapists. The reasons for autism's rise remain unclear. Some experts say the surge in new diagnoses simply reflects better understanding and recognition of the condition, while others suspect that some relatively new environmental factor is causing more children to develop autism. Many parents of autistic children have argued that childhood vaccines cause the condition. But so far, several major scientific studies have failed to find a conclusive link.

The condition's signature disabilities—including difficulties with speech and communication, problems interacting with others, and repetitive behavior—typically appear by an affected child's third birthday. Some forms of autistic disorder cause less severe difficulties, such as trouble making eye contact or holding a long conversation with others. Other forms lead to severe disability, with some children withdrawing from the world around them and avoiding almost all interaction—even a hug from Mom or Dad. Boys develop autism far more often than girls, outnumbering girls in many care settings by three or four to one. While many children respond well to treatment and educational or behavioral therapy, especially if their condition is caught early, there is currently no cure for autism, and an autistic child must continue to live with the disorder as an adult.

The word autism is used very broadly, but actual autism is only one of five related conditions called Pervasive Development Disorders, or PDD:

- **Autistic disorder.** This condition is what most people think of when they think of autism. It is marked by impaired social interaction and communication; delayed speech, social interaction, or play; repetitive or inflexible behavior, with symptoms appearing before the age of three.
- **Asperger's syndrome.** This condition is usually diagnosed later than autism, often in late childhood. Compared to people with other forms of PDD, who often show some level of mental retardation, children with this syndrome often have a normal or high level of intelligence, but they often have trouble connecting with other people. People with Asperger's syndrome often have difficulty with social relationships and making friends, poor physical coordination, and a very narrow, rigid range of interests.
- **Childhood disintegrative disorder.** Children with this condition usually appear to develop normally until their second birthday, babbling, talking, pointing, and playing. Then, between the ages of 2 and 10, they lose some of these important language, social, or physical skills. Instead, they begin to show behaviors and patterns of interaction usually associated with autism—impaired social interaction and communication, and/or repetitive, inflexible behavior.

- **Rett syndrome.** This rare form of PDD is unusual in that it mostly affects girls. Children with this syndrome appear to develop normally for their first six months, but later develop difficulty with talking, major movements such as walking, using their hands, and interacting with other people. In some children with Rett syndrome, these skills never develop normally, while in others, they disappear after first seeming to develop normally.
- **PDD—not otherwise specified.** This category is used to describe children who show some of the symptoms described above, but don't have a large number of them, or only have mild forms of them. These children clearly show some disability, but nothing clear or severe enough to diagnose them with one of the other forms of PDD.

Extensive studies have shown that children with autism have abnormal brain activity, chemistry, and development. Many children with autism also suffer from chronic digestive trouble. Scientists are trying to find what outside factors might help trigger these physical problems, but genes are also increasingly fingered as a culprit in many cases of autism.

How Genes Are Involved

Studies of families with autism first revealed a genetic connection more than 30 years ago. Studies of identical twins have found that if one twin has autism, the other's likelihood of developing the condition ranges anywhere from 60 to more than 90 percent. While fraternal twins or siblings of an autistic child are less likely to share the condition, their risk for autism is still about 75 percent higher than that of the general population—a clear sign that genes factor into the condition.

About 10 percent of autism and PDD cases can be pinned directly to known genes or genetic syndromes, such as the genetic developmental disorder Fragile X syndrome. Rett syndrome is now known to be caused by variations in the *MECP2* gene, also found on the X chromosome. But in the majority of autism and other PDD cases, scientists are still piecing together the many genes and SNPs that appear to play a role. Genes and SNPs that appear related to the condition have been found in many spots on the human genome, including Chromosomes 3, 7, 15, and 17. The exact roles and influences of these genes and SNPs, however, remain unclear. Scientists now believe that multiple genes contribute to autism, and that different genes may also be responsible for different varieties of PDD.

Genetic Testing for Autism

There is currently no single genetic test available for many forms of autism. Scientists do not yet understand autism genetics well enough to be able to offer gene or SNP tests widely.

If you have a child who has already been diagnosed with autism or another form of PDD, however, it's likely that your doctor will recommend genetic testing to see if the condition has been caused by genetic variations such as those responsible for Fragile X or Rett syndromes. This information not only helps clarify the cause of your child's condition, but it also reveals if other children in the family might also be at increased risk. A genetic counselor who specializes in autism, PDD, and other developmental disorders will be able to help you understand your testing options and what a test means for each member of your family.

Special Considerations for Autism and PDD

In their emergence as notable childhood disabilities, autism and PDD have received a great deal of public attention in recent years, mostly due to the efforts of vocal, concerned parents who want a better understanding of the condition and more help for their children. Many of the leaders of this public campaign come from relatively affluent backgrounds, leading to the impression that autism is primarily a problem of white middle-class Americans. This could not be further from the truth. Autism and PDD affect children of all racial groups, ethnic backgrounds, and social classes. Researchers have noted that fewer Latino families report having a child with autism, but they believe this difference may be due to a lack of awareness of the condition, as well as cultural differences that make some families reluctant to label their child as disabled. If you notice unusual behaviors or developmental problems in your child, seek prompt medical attention, no matter your ethnic or class background.

How You Can Treat Autism

Behavioral and educational therapies that help children with autism and PDD interact more comfortably with the world around them often require complex, time-consuming work every day. But, according to many families caring for children with autistic disorders, these interventions have worked wonders. The key, doctors stress, is early diagnosis. You are the best judge of your child's behavior, development, and social skills. If you notice anything that concerns you, talk to your doctor promptly.

Did You Know ?

Serious research into autism isn't limited to vaccines or treatments. Several major universities and research centers have joined the Autism Consortium Gene Discovery Project. This collaborative effort aims to definitively identify all the genes involved in autism and pinpoint their functions. The research relies on about 3,700 DNA samples provided by the Autism Genetic Resource Exchange, a DNA repository for families affected by the condition. This joining of forces between large groups of affected families and scientists represents a significant step toward nailing down how genes drive this condition.

Through special classes, schools, and behavioral therapy at home, even at a very young age, children with autism or other forms of PDD can often make huge improvements. And by entering a network of specialists and other families with similar children, you'll usually find resources that help you as well, making it easier to care for your child and helping everyone in your family.

DOWN SYNDROME

This condition, marked by a combination of physical and mental challenges, involves both mental and physical challenges. Starting in infancy, people with Down syndrome have some degree of developmental and learning disability, along with characteristic facial features, and possible health problems such as heart defects or poor hearing and vision. One of the most common gene-based birth defects, Down syndrome affects 1 in 733 newborns, and patient support groups estimate that about 350,000 Americans have the condition. Down syndrome affects children of all races, ethnic backgrounds, and classes.

The severity of disability in people with Down syndrome varies widely. While the condition commonly creates limitations, improved understanding and therapies now allow a growing number of people with Down syndrome to graduate from high school, hold jobs, and live on their own.

How Genes Are Involved

Down syndrome always starts in the genes, but it is seldom passed on through multiple generations of the same family, unless a person with Down syndrome decides to have a child. Instead, Down syndrome occurs when the cells that create a healthy woman's eggs fail to divide normally. In most cases of Down syndrome, this irregular cell division creates an egg with an extra copy of Chromosome 21. This division error results in an embryo with three copies of the chromosome, a condition formally known as Trisomy 21. In a few cases, Down syndrome also arises from other abnormalities in how Chromosome 21 forms in an embryo. Scientists are still working to determine exactly how this extra or abnormal copy of Chromosome 21 results in the range of birth defects seen in Down syndrome.

Scientists are also trying to determine the cause of the irregular cell division that leads to this chromosomal irregularity. So far, the clearest risks for such problems with Chromosome 21 appear in older mothers. A woman's risk of having a baby with Down syndrome rises sharply with age. A 35-year-old woman, for example, has about a 1 in 350 chance of having a baby with Down syndrome. By the time she is 45, that risk climbs to 1 in 30.

While Down syndrome risks are higher for older mothers, age alone can't prevent the condition. About 80 percent of babies with Down syndrome are born to women under the age of 35. This number reflects the fact that younger mothers have the majority of babies, and until recently, usually didn't receive the same level of Down syndrome screening during pregnancy as older women.

Genetic Testing for Down Syndrome

Unless your doctor thinks there is some reason you may be at special risk, there is no test routinely offered prior to a pregnancy to see if would-be parents are at greater genetic risk of having a baby with Down syndrome. If you are newly pregnant, however, genetic tests to check your developing baby for Down syndrome are widely available. You can choose from a range of options, including blood tests that are less invasive but also less reliable than other options, a more reliable combination of a blood test and a special ultrasound scan, or a highly accurate but more invasive test that analyzes fetal chromosomes using samples of tissue or amniotic fluid. (For more information on prenatal testing, see Chapter 3.)

Until recently, more reliable forms of Down syndrome screening were only offered to expectant mothers over the age of 35. But revised medical recommendations issued in 2006 now make it easier for pregnant women of any age to receive thorough Down syndrome screening, making testing for all mothers a routine part of pregnancy and making it more likely that insurance coverage will pay the cost. (For more information on the recommendations, see Chapter 3.) Some families who find that their developing baby has Down syndrome use the information to help them better prepare for their child's special needs after birth. Others decide to end the pregnancy.

Testing is also possible once a baby is born. If you give birth to a baby suspected of having Down syndrome, your doctor will recommend a genetic test to study the baby's chromosomes and confirm the diagnosis.

A Shorter Wait for Down Syndrome Results

For many years, expectant mothers who underwent fetal diagnostic screening for Down syndrome had to endure more than a week of waiting to learn their test results. Fortunately, a newer analysis technique, called FISH, makes it possible to get a preliminary result in just a few days. FISH, or fluorescent *in situ* hybridization, makes it possible to analyze fetal DNA much more quickly than a regular test. Your FISH test won't provide as much information as your full amniocentesis or CVS test result, but it can offer basic results. A FISH test often costs an additional $200 or more, however, and may not be covered by your insurance. If you are considering a FISH test, check with your insurance company ahead of time. (For more information on prenatal testing, see Chapter 3.)

Special Considerations for Down Syndrome

Many expectant mothers, especially younger women, welcome the broader approach to Down syndrome testing. But some families of children with Down syndrome are less sure. They see their children as valuable members of society with unique insights to offer and lessons to share. Wider testing, they say, will result in more abortions in Down syndrome pregnancies and fewer Down syndrome children living among us.

If you are pregnant and found to be carrying a Down syndrome baby, your genetic counselor will help you consider all your options. Some families are not willing or prepared to raise a baby with Down syndrome. Others are more open to the idea, or have religious or ethical beliefs that do not support abortions. Your counselor and doctor can help you make the right decision for your family.

How You Can Treat Down Syndrome

There is no cure for the condition, but parents of children with Down syndrome rarely have to face the challenges of raising their child alone. Many special education programs are available to help children with Down syndrome make their way through school and learn to interact with others. While some children with the condition attend special schools or classes, a growing number of children with Down syndrome attend regular schools alongside other children. Doctors who specialize in Down syndrome help with the condition's physical effects. And support groups aid families in providing the best possible care for children with Down syndrome. Treatment and development plans for Down syndrome are as individual as each child born with the condition. By building a supportive network of doctors, teachers, therapists, and other Down syndrome families, you can create an approach uniquely tailored to your child.

FRAGILE X SYNDROME

Fragile X syndrome is the most common form of inherited mental disorder. The condition is marked by delayed mental and physical development and learning disabilities. Fragile X usually also brings behaviors and aversions similar to autism. Children with Fragile X tend to have shorter attention spans, and they may easily become overwhelmed by what is going on around them. Prone to being anxious, these children often exhibit unusual or repetitive behaviors, such as flapping or biting their hands. Children with Fragile X also sometimes develop seizures and are more prone to ear infections, poor vision, and digestive problems.

The condition affects boys more profoundly, both in terms of numbers and severity. As its name suggests, Fragile X affects the X chromosome, making it a sex-linked disorder with especially serious effects in boys. Fragile X syndrome appears in about 1 in every 4,000 boys, compared to 1 in every 8,000 girls. The condition is found in children of all ethnic backgrounds. Some children with the condition don't look physically different from other people. But many, especially boys, develop a long, narrow face, large ears, and/or overly flexible joints. While most boys with Fragile X have significant mental impairment or learning disabilities, only about one-half to one-third of affected girls do. Girls with Fragile X are also less likely to have any physical signs of their condition. (For more information on sex-linked genetic disorders, see Chapter 1.)

How Genes are Involved

Fragile X syndrome is caused by a variation in a gene on the X chromosome called *FMR1*. Exactly how this genetic difference causes the development of Fragile X isn't yet clear, but scientists do know how to recognize it. In Fragile X, a particular section of bases that spell out part of the gene is repeated too many times. While it is normal for most people to have a few such repeats in this gene, too many repeats shut the gene down. Under a microscope, the gene repeats also make the affected section of the X chromosome look thin or flimsy, hence the condition's name. This type of abnormality in the number of bases in a particular spot on the genome is called a copy number variant, a growing focus of medical genomics that is examined more closely in Chapter 9.

As a sex-linked disorder, Fragile X syndrome is usually passed on by a mother who is a carrier. A woman is considered a carrier of Fragile X if she either has 60 to 200 repeats within her *FMR1* gene, a condition called a pre-mutation, or more than 200 repeats, which add up to a full mutation. While a pre-mutation often doesn't cause symptoms of Fragile X syndrome, the number of repeats sometimes expands while the *FMR1* gene is being copied and passed from mother to child, making it possible for a pre-mutation carrier to have a child with a full mutation. Men with a pre-mutation can also pass it on to their daughters, making them carriers. (For more information about how sex-linked disorders are passed between parents and children, see Chapter 1).

> *Did You Know* ?
>
> As gene-screening technology improves and drops in cost, more newborn boys may someday be screened for Fragile X syndrome. The condition is common enough to make universal testing worthwhile, some gene experts say, because children benefit more from treatment if their condition is caught early. Right now, most children aren't diagnosed until after their second birthday.
>
> Other doctors and insurance companies, however, say Fragile X testing remains too complex and expensive to justify more widespread screening. But if the costs for this type of DNA analysis drop, expect to see more childhood development experts push for widespread screening for baby boys.

Genetic Testing for Fragile X

Genetic testing is available to look for *FMR1* variations and pre-mutations. The test is not commonly offered as part of pre-pregnancy or prenatal carrier testing for most people. But if Fragile X or mental and developmental disability of unknown cause run in your family, your doctor will likely recommend a genetic test if you are planning a pregnancy or are already expecting. (For more information on genetic testing and pregnancy, see Chapter 3.)

Children with signs of mental or developmental delays or autism are often offered genetic testing to see if their condition can be pinned on a Fragile X variation. If genetic testing uncovers a Fragile X variation in your child, this information can help guide treatment decisions and help shape any plans you may have for future children.

Special Considerations for Fragile X Syndrome

While prenatal genetic testing can tell you whether your developing baby carries a Fragile X variation, it can't always reveal your child's fate. While most boys with Fragile X have serious learning or mental disabilities, many girls with a Fragile X variation do not, as their other X chromosome protects them. Girls with a Fragile X variation often experience fewer or less severe mental and learning disabilities than boys with Fragile X syndrome. Talk to a genetic counselor who specializes in developmental disabilities about what test results might mean for your baby before and after undergoing any Fragile X testing.

How You Can Treat Fragile X Syndrome

There is no cure for Fragile X, but early educational and behavioral therapies, often starting while your child is still a toddler, can greatly improve many aspects of your child's life, including speech, anxiousness, and learning skills. Children with more serious health problems caused by Fragile X, such as seizures, are usually treated with medication.

FREQUENTLY ASKED QUESTIONS ABOUT GENES, THE BRAIN AND MENTAL HEALTH

Q. A few years ago, it seemed like childhood vaccines were debated as a main cause of autism. Now, doctors usually say that vaccines don't cause autism, and that genes probably play a significant role. I'm not sure what to think. It sounds like doctors just want to defend vaccines no matter what and are trying to put the blame for autism on parents and their genes instead. What's really behind this change?

A. The shift reflects a lot of scientific research into both vaccines and autism genes. It's true that many parents with autistic children wonder if vaccines contributed to their children's problem, and some are waging legal challenges against vaccine makers. But major scientific studies looking into vaccines and autism have failed to find a connection. At the same time, research into autism genes has improved. The role of genes in autism, though, doesn't mean that parents are somehow to blame for their children's condition. And so far, known autism genes only increase a child's risk for the disorder. As with many of these complex conditions, it probably takes a combination of genetic and environmental factors working together to cause the condition to surface. External factors—perhaps a medication, a food, or a virus—may play a role in causing autism when paired with a genetic predisposition. Many scientists and millions of dollars are now at work deciphering what really drives this condition.

Q. *I think it's really arrogant of some health experts to be so reluctant to let people use the* APOE e4 *test for Alzheimer's risk. In recommending against this test, they say they are concerned about people's well-being. Well, so am I—my own! Two of my relatives developed Alzheimer's in their 70s. I want to know if I'm at a higher risk. Why can't doctors let me make up my own mind?*

A. The recommendations against the *APOE e4* test stem from the fact that there isn't much you can yet do with a positive test result. If your test shows you're at a higher risk, that's no guarantee you'll develop Alzheimer's disease. And in the meantime, relatively little is known about how to prevent and treat the disease. The test may give you worrisome information that you can't act on. If you feel strongly about being tested, though, talk to your doctor and/or a genetic counselor. If you remain interested in the test, and your doctor believes you understand all the ramifications, there's a better chance he'll support your decision. If you would prefer to be tested on your own, several Web-based genetic firms now offer that option. If you go that route, however, consider choosing a company that also offers genetic counseling, so that you aren't left to interpret your results alone. And remember that, over time, this dilemma is likely to change. Many doctors say they'll be more enthusiastic about the *APOE e4* test when more is known about preventing and treating Alzheimer's disease.

Q. *When it comes to bad behavior and alcoholism, my family tree is a pretty scary place. We have alcoholics on both sides of the family, a few of whom drank themselves to death. I don't drink much myself, but sometimes I wonder if it's only a matter of time before the family drinking gene turns on in my head and gets me into trouble. What can I do to make sure I don't wind up like some of my relatives?*

A. Start by acknowledging all the factors in your favor—including your desire to follow a different path. So far, genes linked to addiction or alcoholism only appear to increase risk. It's unlikely a single gene will suddenly compel you to start drinking heavily. And your family's drinking pattern could be a habit learned from generation to generation, rather than a reflection of any gene. So far, you've taken the most important step you can to protect yourself—you're aware of your risk and want to do something about it. Be watchful of any changes in your drinking habits, or any tendency toward reaching for alcohol or any addictive substance during stressful times. Get in touch with groups such as Adult Children of Alcoholics, which provide community meetings, valuable information, and support. Along with your genes, an important force in protecting your health is your power to choose. By deciding you'd like to follow a route different from your family's, you are off to a great beginning.

Q. *I had to take a couple of different antidepressants before I found the right one, and the genetic test to help choose the right medicine is great news. But why don't insurance companies always want to pay for the test? You'd think they'd be happy to pay, since it would mean fewer problems and doctor visits while people try to find the best antidepressant.*

A. Limited insurance coverage for these tests reflects how new they are, as well as lingering questions about how much they help. The CYP450 and *5-HTT* tests can't tell you which antidepressant will help you most, only which ones probably won't help. It's still possible to take these genetic tests and wind up trying more than one antidepressant. There's also the issue of cost. Worldwide, drug companies sell about $20 billion worth of antidepressants each year—a figure that reflects tens of millions of prescriptions. Each of these genetic tests costs hundreds of dollars, and if each person using an antidepressant took them, the costs to insurance companies would skyrocket. As the tests become more precise, however, and their costs come down, it's more likely that insurance will cover more of their cost.

Q. *I have a little girl with mild Down syndrome, and she loves school and reading and learning. I feel confident that she'll finish high school and probably find a job. But what about the emotional aspects of her life when she grows up? What if she wants to get married and have children? Would her children have Down syndrome, as well?*

A. Many people with Down syndrome are happily married. The issue of children, though, raises complicated questions that require a lot of thought and sensitive counseling. Only about half of women with Down syndrome are fertile, and those who are face a higher risk of miscarriage. Between 35 and 50 percent of children born to mothers with Down syndrome will share their mother's condition or have another developmental disability. And the costs of raising children can be especially hard for a Down syndrome parent with more limited career opportunities. If your daughter is interested in having children later on, she'll need lots of support in making that decision.

KEEP IN MIND

Your genes build your brain and its basic functions—including your brain cells and how they communicate to handle the complicated work they do.

These genes have plenty of influence over how your brain works, how you think, and even how you feel. If a particular mental health issue or neurological illness runs in your family, you may be at a higher risk for the same problem yourself. But as with other parts of your body, the genes linked to your brain usually don't work alone. Outside influences—such as habits learned from your family, an acquired illness, even your diet—also affect your mood, thoughts, and behavior.

Because the power of so many of these genes is limited, current genetic tests for many mental health and neurological problems often aren't conclusive. While genetic tests are reliable for completely DNA-driven conditions such as Down syndrome, tests for issues such as your response to certain antidepressants often point out the likelihood of a problem, but not the certainty of one. While this information can sometimes be helpful, it's not the same thing as a definitive answer.

The limits to genes that shape your brain and personality, however, also offer a priceless opportunity. Through your surroundings and the choices you make, you have plenty of say over how your brain works, your behavior, and your mental health.

Given everything we still don't know about genes and the brain, the study of how DNA affects behavior and mental health remains one of the most cutting-edge aspects of genomic science. The implications of behavioral genetics also raise broader concerns that apply to every aspect of genomic understanding. In this new era of personal genetic knowledge, how will your genetic privacy be protected? Could your DNA information be used against you? Could understanding your DNA put you at risk for discrimination? These questions are common, but new options also make them less worrisome. We'll look at these issues, some of the most important in genomic care, next.

CHAPTER EIGHT

PROTECTING YOUR GENOMIC PRIVACY

Heidi Williams was well schooled in the fortunate difference distinguishing her two children from her. The young mother from Cecilia, Kentucky, suffers from a genetic disorder called alpha 1 antitrypsin deficiency, or AAT, which has left her without enough of a key protein that maintains healthy liver and lung function. Heidi knew her condition required regular care. But she took some comfort in the fact that her two children, Jayme and Jesse, were only carriers of her AAT mutation. Each had inherited a copy of the mutation, but that single copy would never cause either of them to share their mother's illness.

When Heidi went searching for health coverage for her children, however, she learned that insurance decision-makers aren't always so well informed about genetics.

Heidi called Humana, Inc., a major insurance provider, to seek insurance in August 2003. A company representative first seemed eager to cover the children, offering a policy for $105 per month. Then the representative started to walk Heidi through the application process, asking for details of the family medical history. Heidi, following laws that require truthful disclosure of any noteworthy medical issues, told the representative about her children's AAT carrier status.

The application then hit a wall. Humana supervisors joined the discussion. Heidi kept repeating that the children were only carriers who would never get sick from their mutation. Her assurances did no good.

A week later, Heidi received a letter from Humana, denying her children health insurance because of their carrier status. And, Heidi discovered, she had no legal grounds to complain. At that time, a gap in federal law left people like her searching for coverage on the individual insurance market, vulnerable to rejection for genetic reasons.

But Heidi was angry enough to keep pressing her case, even if the law didn't back her up. She sought the help of other families with the same AAT mutation. She gathered the support of a prominent genetic fairness advocacy group, a law firm, and a leading AAT physician. She sent Humana an appeal, backed by letters and stacks of evidence supporting her assertion of the children's good health. The company turned her children down again.

Only after the media learned of her fight and began questioning Humana did the company relent and offer the children insurance in the spring of 2004. By that time, Heidi had found coverage elsewhere. While she said "No" to Humana, she was pleased the company had changed its position. But she couldn't help but wonder whether the episode was a preview of her children's future.

"No one should have to force an insurance company to cover perfectly healthy children," she later told a federal advisory committee studying genetic discrimination. "In fact, I don't believe it should have mattered what their genetic status was to begin with.

"I should not have had to spend six months wondering if the decision to have my children's genetic status verified by their pediatrician was a huge mistake," Heidi said in her testimony before the committee. "I should not have to wonder if my children's genetic status is going to follow them into the work force.... And I certainly should not have to feel guilty for passing this genetic anomaly on to my children."

Heidi's experience with genetic misunderstanding helped drive passage of one of the most important legal changes in the world of genomics—a 2008 federal law prohibiting many forms of genetic discrimination. The Genetic Information Nondiscrimination Act (GINA) bars genetic bias in health insurance and employment decisions. While the law doesn't cover every possible use of your genetic information, it takes an important step towards a society in which DNA is no basis for discrimination. In this chapter, you'll learn about GINA and other legal tools that help you to protect your genomic privacy and guard against bias.

ETHICAL, LEGAL AND SOCIAL IMPLICATIONS OF GENETICS

The information contained in your DNA is often of great interest to others—relatives, government officials, your insurance company, and scientific researchers. But their interest may not always be to your benefit. Gene experts sum up these competing concerns as the ethical, legal, and social implications (or ELSI) of human genomics.

Ethical questions are so intertwined with genomic medicine that we address them throughout this book. But you also have many other issues to consider, ranging from family privacy to health coverage. To get a better sense of the complex questions you might face in your genomic-driven care, consider the following situations that gene experts face every day in helping patients:

- If people in a particular population group carry a certain risk-related mutation, will the whole community face systematic bias or stigma from certain types of insurance companies, such as life insurers?
- Given the high costs of many forms of genomic medicine, how can society help those with low incomes benefit from genomic advances?

- If you donate DNA for research, and a scientist makes an important discovery as a result, who should own that discovery—you, the scientist, or humanity at large? Should anyone be able to make money from it?

Public opinion polls have repeatedly reflected a strong desire for genetic privacy and strong anti-discrimination laws. The passage of GINA takes a major step toward addressing those concerns, with the law's health insurance protections taking effect in May 2009 and the employment protections taking effect in November 2009. While these protections have not been tested in the judicial system, advocates for the law say that most Americans can now feel safe from genetic discrimination in health insurance and employment.

While GINA is powerful, however, it isn't comprehensive. A few other types of health-related insurance, such as life insurance, aren't covered by the law. A few sectors of society, such as the military, are exempt. In such situations, there are important steps you can take to assess your own risks and determine what legal protections may be available. In this book, we can't offer you definitive medical or legal advice. But we can give you a better idea of how to protect your genetic information and what situations require you to ask tough questions.

LAWS CONTROLLING THE USE OF DNA INFORMATION

HIPAA

Before GINA, a powerful national law already existed that protected you from some invasions of genomic privacy and genomic discrimination. The federal Health Insurance Portability and Accountability Act (HIPAA) was passed in 1996 and protects patient privacy in many of the most common health care settings. HIPAA prohibits most health care providers and health plans—such as doctors, hospitals, group health plans, and health maintenance organizations (HMO)—from indiscriminately sharing or disclosing a patient's medical records. Upon GINA's passage, HIPAA was amended to explicitly state that genetic information should be considered medical information and receive the same privacy protections.

HIPAA requires health care providers to obtain your consent before they share your information for purposes related to medical care, such as treatment, insurance coverage, and billing. When your doctor's office or hospital asks you to sign forms that explain how your medical information will be used and shared, they are following HIPAA guidelines.

In a few instances, such as when a relative's health is in jeopardy or police or judges demand your information, your medical and gene information can be shared without your permission. But in most cases, health care providers covered by HIPAA may not share medical information widely. Your family doctor, for example, cannot call your child's teacher to reveal details of any recent medical or genetic test your child recently underwent.

The federal HIPAA law prohibits discrimination only in some cases. HIPAA does offer broad anti-bias protections if you are part of a commercially issued group health plan. If your employer, for example, contracts with an HMO or PPO (preferred provider organization) to provide employee health insurance, HIPAA safeguards cover that plan. HIPAA prevents group health plans from using any health factor, including genetic information, as a basis for limiting, denying, or charging more for coverage. If your gene information shows that you are at increased risk for a particular illness, HIPAA also offers you an important protection. The law specifically states that genetic information in the absence of illness shall not be considered a pre-existing condition.

Limits of HIPAA

Some types of insurance providers, including worker's compensation, life, and disability insurers, are not covered by many medical privacy laws, and may request and handle your medical or genomic information more freely. In these types of insurance, insurers may also ask for family history and use the information to decide on coverage.

The same is true of many medical and genetic researchers, who may store your gene information for scientific study. While many scientists are conscientious and follow the confidentiality rules established by

A DOCTOR'S DECISION

Courts Say Physicians Have a "Duty to Warn" At-Risk Relatives

Safer v. Pack

If you or someone in your family has a genetic condition, the doctor handling the case is legally obligated to inform you or your relatives. In 1996, an important court decision spelled out a physician's "duty to warn" in genetic cases—including taking "reasonable steps" to share that warning with a patient's family if necessary.

The case, *Safer v. Pack*, arose after Donna Safer, then 36, was diagnosed with colon cancer as a result of an inherited predisposition mutation. Her father had died at the age of 45. At the time, his physician, Dr. George Pack, only told the family that Mr. Safer had died of a vaguely defined cause. After digging into her father's medical records after her own diagnosis, Safer discovered he had also been diagnosed with colon cancer. She sued Pack's estate, saying the doctor had failed to warn her family.

An appeals court agreed with Safer, ruling that a doctor has a "duty to warn those known to be at risk of avoidable harm from a genetically transmissible condition." Federal medical privacy laws contain provisions allowing doctors to offer such warnings to relatives.

scientific oversight boards, most researchers are not covered by HIPAA. However, in response to concerns from research participants, many genetic research studies have applied for and received Certificates of Confidentiality, which are issued by the Department of Health and Human Services and offer an additional layer of protection from third parties who might want access to genetic information.

Many direct-to-consumer medical information and testing companies are not required to follow HIPAA rules. While these companies handle health-related information, most opened their doors after HIPAA was crafted and do not fall under the law's control. Some, however, still choose to follow HIPAA standards. Ask any genetic testing company you might work with about whether or not the firm is HIPAA-consistent.

GINA

After 13 years in development, GINA provides a national baseline against genetic discrimination in decisions about health insurance. GINA strictly prohibits:

- Health insurers from requiring individuals to provide personal or family members' genetic information to the insurer for eligibility, coverage, underwriting, or to set premiums.
- Health insurers from using genetic information to make enrollment or coverage decisions.
- Health insurers from requesting or requiring an individual or an individual's family member to undergo a genetic test.
- Using genetic information as a pre-existing condition in the Medicare supplemental policy and individual health insurance markets.

If you are submitting claims for health management options that result from a genetic test result, the insurer may request genetic information. For example, women with an increased risk of breast cancer because of a *BRCA* gene mutation would begin having screening mammograms and MRIs at age 25, and the insurer can request information about her mutation status prior to authorizing payment.

Limits of GINA

GINA is not a panacea. The law does not include protections from genetic discrimination when obtaining life, disability, or long-term care insurance. It is also important to remember that GINA specifically protects people who do not yet have symptoms of a DNA-related condition, so it does not protect people who have already developed early signs of a genetic disease. If you have already developed an illness, however, you may be protected by HIPAA. GINA does not apply to employers with fewer than 15 employees or to members of the U.S. military.

Weighing the Pros and Cons of Genetic Testing

In 1998, Steve, the proud father of four daughters, discovered that his mother had a BRCA1 mutation. During his initial genetic counseling session, he learned that as a male, his chances of developing cancer were low, even if he carried the same predisposition mutation. However, his daughters would be at an increased risk if they were to inherit the mutation from him. During that session, Steve declined genetic testing, stating his concern that his girls would face genetic discrimination in the future if he carried the mutation.

In 2003, however, when his oldest daughter was 25, we revisited the issue of testing. If he were to have a mutation (and he had a 50 percent chance of having one) *and* his daughter were to have a mutation (another 50 percent), we would recommend that she begin having mammograms and breast MRIs that year. But Steve was still reluctant to have testing. Further counseling revealed that he was terrified to pass his mutation to his girls. He had felt helpless as he watched so many of the women in his family battle cancer. In the last 10 years, his mother had died of ovarian cancer, and two of his sisters still battled breast cancer. As tears rolled down his cheeks, he acknowledged that he was terrified of passing this deadly mutation on to his four little princesses.

During our counseling sessions, we balance patient concerns about genetic discrimination with the potential value of knowing their genetic information. In Steve's case, it was only when his daughters reached age 25 that this genetic information would have affected how they managed their health care.

Meanwhile, in 2002, legislators in Steve's home state of Utah passed a law to guard against genetic discrimination. The law defines what is considered private genetic information and outlines both the use and access restrictions on employers and health insurers. It also lays out the rights and enforcement options for people who feel they are the victims of genetic discrimination.

Though still anxious, Steve decided to have testing. Steve and his wife agreed that they did not want to compromise their daughters' ability to make health care decisions. Thankfully, the results showed that he didn't have the mutation. Both he and his wife shed tears of joy when they heard the news. His wife wished he had been tested five years earlier to spare them the years of worrying, but before this new law was passed, Steve had simply been too concerned about discrimination. And once the law was in place, he then faced his fear of passing the mutation to his girls before agreeing to the test.

Bottom Line: As a genetic counselor, I am thrilled that the passage of GINA has provided national protection. In the past, I often found myself reassuring our patients about their genetic discrimination concerns. Now, the risks of discrimination are much lower, and I am happy to find myself counseling patients more about concerns of real importance to their health, and less about fears of possible bias.

Additional State Protections

Most states have passed additional genetic privacy and anti-dis-crimination laws of their own. These regulations vary widely from state to state. For example, at least five states, including Alaska, Colorado, Florida, Georgia, and Louisiana, have explicitly defined genetic infor-mation as personal property. Other states, however, have made no such legal distinction over ownership of genetic information.

In the realm of life, disability, and long-term care insurance, the only anti-discrimination safeguards are those passed by individual states. Again, these vary widely from state to state. More than a dozen states restrict genetic discrimination in life insurance or disability insurance, and about 10 prohibit genetic discrimination in long-term care coverage. In most cases, the safeguards in GINA are stronger than those that were initially determined by state laws. In those cases, GINA provides the baseline protection. However, if a state's law is stronger and provides more protections than GINA, that part of the state law will trump.

PROTECTING YOUR PRIVACY

Since HIPAA covers your medical information, including your genomic data, you can guard your privacy by following some basic medical confidentiality guidelines created by groups such as the Health Privacy Project, a non-profit consumer advocacy group:

- Request a copy of your medical record from your health-care providers. Keeping copies of your records lets you see what infor-mation has been documented and how it has been shared.
- Find out if you have a file with the Medical Information Bureau (MIB), and if you do, request a copy. About 20 percent of Americans have a file with this organization made up of about 600 insurers. Insurance companies use MIB to share patient information as they make coverage decisions. According to MIB, these files do not include a person's entire medical record. Instead, they document if a person has a serious health condition that might influence insurance rulings. Go to www.mib.com to find out about getting a copy of your file, or call 866-692-6901. Consumers may receive one copy of their MIB record a year at no charge.
- Talk about confidentiality concerns with your doctor. Find out how his medical practice handles privacy concerns and medical records. Many records, for example, are now outsourced overseas for processing or transcribing. If your records are sent out of the country for handling, ask what privacy protections are in place.
- Read authorization forms before signing and edit them to limit the sharing of information. Not all medical caregivers agree to

allow you to edit these forms, but privacy experts say it's worth making the effort. Take a minute to understand the fine print in privacy disclosures.

- Register objections to disclosures you don't find acceptable. Many health care providers now have a privacy specialist who can take complaints and address concerns in detail.
- Learn about the privacy protections in your state. The National Conference of State Legislatures maintains a thorough overview of laws related to genetic care in each state on its Web site at www.ncsl.org. Even with GINA in place, some states have stronger protections that may benefit you.
- Contact advocacy and support groups that track discrimination laws, privacy rights, and policy changes. They also help consumers get answers to questions on gene-related care. Genetic Alliance, a non-profit group that represents a variety of patient interests, has helped many consumers. They can be found online at www.geneticalliance.org or can be reached by phone at 202-966-5557.
- Be especially cautious when providing personal medical information for surveys, health screenings, and health-related Web sites. Medical privacy laws often do not cover many such organizations.

HOW YOU CAN PROTECT YOUR HEALTH INSURANCE

Given that GINA is in the early stages of implementation, there may still be gaps in legal protections against insurance privacy and discrimination, and insurance industry employees may need time to understand the laws. Therefore, genetic experts suggest the following steps:

- Start by learning your rights in your state and your workplace. Do you live in a state that offers more genetic protections, or fewer, than GINA? Is your health plan covered by HIPAA? Knowing the answers to these questions will give you a better sense of what legal protections you have.
- If your genomic information leads to insurance problems, try the approach used by Heidi Williams. Argue your case, and seek outside help. Insurance companies can sometimes be persuaded to reverse their decisions.
- Some people, reluctant to share their gene information with insurers, may fail to disclose gene-related conditions. But withholding such information constitutes fraud and can create more problems for you later on. If an insurer asks for your genomic information, determine that the insurer has the right to ask for the information and then answer truthfully.
- Be ready to share your genomic know-how with insurance company employees. As Heidi Williams discovered, your insurance

company many not have any idea how to analyze your genomic information correctly. If you encounter an insurance decision-maker who doesn't understand your genomic health issues, seek support from your doctor or genetic counselor, who can back you up with explanations and letters of support. Also, seek direct communication with the medical director of your insurance company, who may understand your information better than other staff members, whose expertise may lie more in business or mathematics.

EMPLOYMENT PROTECTION

Until GINA's passage, employment protections varied as wildly as insurance protections. GINA prohibits many forms of work-related genetic discrimination, and another federal law—the Americans With Disabilities Act (ADA)—helps as well. Some states have also stepped in to provide stronger safeguards against gene-related employment discrimination.

Protecting Genetic Privacy on the Job

Norman-Bloodsaw v. Lawrence Berkeley Laboratories

In 1994, an employee at a major national science center in California looked at a copy of her workplace medical record and saw an unusual string of letters. The letters represented a code for a medical test. Her discovery prompted one of the most significant cases confirming the right of patient privacy in the realm of genetic information.

The employee, Marya Norman-Bloodsaw, worked at Lawrence Berkeley Laboratories (LBL), a federal research facility. The code she spotted on her medical records led her to realize that the lab was testing employees for medical conditions without their knowledge or direct consent. One of those tests, conducted on African-American workers, looked for sickle cell trait, a genetic mutation. The secret testing had been going on for decades.

Norman-Bloodsaw and other employees sued the lab, alleging violations of civil rights and the right to privacy. The lab countered that the workers had agreed to undergo general medical exams. That agreement, the lab said, meant the workers also agreed to the testing done in secret. In 1998, a federal appeals court sided with the workers, saying such tests violate the right to privacy. LBL wound up paying affected employees $2.2 million in an out-of-court settlement.

"The constitutionally protected privacy interest in avoiding disclosure of personal matters clearly encompasses medical information and its confidentiality," the ruling stated. "One can think of few subject areas more personal and more likely to implicate privacy interests than that of one's health or genetic make-up."

The Americans with Disabilities Act

A key law that offers some protections against a worker being fired or demoted because of a genetic condition is the Americans with Disabilities Act, or ADA. This law prohibits job discrimination against those with disabilities, and includes diagnosed, symptomatic genetic illness as a disability. It does not consider carriers or people at a higher genetic risk of disease as disabled, although this interpretation of the law is still not well tested in court. But the ADA has set important legal standards for companies to follow in the genomic realm. In 2001, the U.S. Equal Employment

Lawsuit Affirms Employment Rights

EEOC v. Burlington Northern & Santa Fe R.R. Co.

Painful injuries of the hands, wrists, and forearms—often caused by an inflammatory condition called carpal tunnel syndrome—are a common problem in today's workplaces. They're also expensive cases for companies to treat. But when a Texas-based railroad decided to try a new approach to handling its workers' carpal tunnel complaints, the company launched a major fight over genetics and privacy.

Railway employees who filed claims for work-related carpal tunnel injuries found themselves being forced to give blood samples as part of their claim. A few started asking questions, and learned that each sample was being subjected to a genetic test. The company was looking to see if employees with carpal tunnel claims suffered from a hereditary condition called HNPP, or Hereditary Neuropathy with liability to Pressure Palsies.

Caused by a genetic mutation on Chromosome 17, HNPP is extremely rare. Depending on the population studied, it is estimated that between two and 16 people in 100,000 have HNPP. But a positive gene test might have allowed the railroad to argue that an employee's carpal tunnel case was caused by something other than work-related injury. Until employees uncovered the testing, they'd had no idea the railway was testing them for genetic illness.

Affected employees, together with their union, appealed to federal regulators, saying the testing violated laws that govern when companies can force employees into medical tests. In February 2001, the U.S. Equal Employment Opportunity Commission filed suit against Burlington Northern, saying the testing violated worker protections spelled out in the Americans with Disabilities Act. Thirty employees eventually joined the suit.

Two months later, Burlington Northern settled the case for $2.2 million. The railway also agreed to stop testing its workers, to disregard the results of any tests conducted to date, and not to retaliate against any employee who joined the case. The case, a major test of genetic protections offered by the Americans with Disabilities Act, set an important precedent protecting employees from gene discrimination on the job.

Opportunity Commission used gene-related portions of ADA to file and win an important case against genetic discrimination in the workplace.

GINA and Employment

In addition to addressing health insurance, GINA covers many concerns in the workplace. Specifically, GINA strictly prohibits:

- An employer from using genetic information to make decisions about hiring, promoting, terms or conditions, privileges of employment, compensation, or termination.
- An employer, employment agency, labor organization, or training program from limiting, segregating, or classifying an employee or member, or depriving that employee or member of employment opportunities, on the basis of genetic information.
- An employer, employment agency, labor organization, or training program from requesting, requiring, or purchasing genetic information of the individual or a family member of the individual except in rare cases. The exceptions to this are when the information is inadvertently provided or if the information is publicly available.
- An employment agency, labor organization, or training program from failing or refusing to refer an individual for employment on the basis of genetic information.
- An employer, labor organization, or joint labor/management committee from using genetic information to make decisions regarding admission to or employment in any program for apprenticeship or training and retraining, including on-the-job training.
- A labor organization from excluding or expelling from membership, or otherwise discriminating against, an individual because of genetic information.

Additional State Protections

Many states have passed their own laws, although these vary widely in scope and strength. More than 30 states have laws prohibiting discrimination in hiring, firing, or setting the terms of employment. Employers are prohibited from requiring genetic testing or genetic information in about 25 states, and from performing genetic tests in more than 15.

WHO OWNS YOUR GENOME?

If you were to donate a sample of your DNA for scientific research, you'd find the medical side of the process very similar to that of giving DNA for a medical test. You'd sign a consent form and most likely have blood drawn. But once your DNA sample heads to the lab, the similarity ends.

When you give a DNA sample for a medical test, the analysis is being performed solely for your benefit. You give permission for the test and are informed of its results. But when you donate DNA for science, you are, in many cases, giving your genetic information away. There is no one standard set of rules that governs how gene researchers must handle samples or interact with the people who donated them. If a mutation that has clinical consequences is found, some research projects are designed to inform you. Others cannot.

And what happens when an important discovery is made using your genes? Again, the answers vary widely. Some research projects, especially those funded with public money, make their scientific results available to other researchers for free. In these projects, the findings from your DNA become the property of humanity, available to benefit anyone. Other researchers, however, may try to turn gene discoveries into profit, by saying that they hold exclusive rights to their findings and turning them into money-making tests or treatments.

This practice is known as gene patenting, in which genes are patented

IN THE NEWS

A Family Fights Gene Patenting

Greenberg et al v. Miami Children's Hospital Research Institute

If you think gene patents sound more like science fiction than real life, talk to Dan and Debbie Greenberg. They gave scientists their DNA to try to stop a deadly genetic disease, only to wind up seeing their donation used for profit.

In the 1980s, the Greenbergs lost two of their children to Canavan disease, an incurable genetic brain disorder. Canavan disease arises from a recessive mutation on Chromosome 17, and almost all cases occur in Jews of European descent. While the disease is very rare, it is also devastating, destroying the brain and causing death in the first years of life.

When the Greenbergs lost their children, doctors had no carrier test to offer would-be parents at risk for the Canavan mutation. The Greenbergs, working with other Jewish families and genetic health organizations, decided to change that. They found a scientist willing to search for the Canavan gene, and donated DNA, tissue, and money to start the research. In 1997, the scientist, then working at Miami Children's Hospital, found the Canavan gene. A carrier test quickly followed—as did a patent.

The Greenbergs thought this discovery would be widely available throughout the Jewish community. They were stunned and angry when the hospital began aggressively enforcing the patent, demanding royalties for the test and limiting the number of labs that could perform the test. In 2000, the Greenbergs and community groups sued the hospital and its researchers. The patent and commercial test, they said, would mean fewer people could use the test, and that future Canavan research would be limited.

The case settled in 2003. While the terms of the deal remain confidential, some details were spelled out. The hospital kept its patent, but the Canavan gene can now be used freely in research trying to cure the disease.

just the same as any other invention. The rules for gene patents were first spelled out in a set of guidelines issued by U.S. government officials in 2001. Under the rules, no one can patent the entire human genome. But individual human genes can be patented, giving the patent holder exclusive rights over their use. There are more than 6,000 such patents on file.

Many scientists and companies say such patents are fair and necessary. A gene patent is the only way to give investors in genomic research a return on their investment. But critics say gene patenting is wrong. Claiming ownership over fundamental instructions for human life is unethical, they say. A gene patent can potentially hurt patients with a genetic condition, by blocking further research or medical care involving that gene, or by significantly limiting access to testing by making it expensive.

Protecting Your Information in Research Studies

Getting answers to a few questions before you join any genomic research study can help you avoid later surprises:

- Know exactly how your DNA will be handled and used.
- Get a clear understanding of the intention of the research. Is it intended to create medical treatments for a profit?
- Ask how your privacy will be protected.
- Ask if you'll be informed of any significant discoveries found in your DNA or made using your DNA.
- Know who will own those discoveries and who will benefit from them.

Answers to these questions should be spelled out in the consent form the research project staff asks you to sign. If they are not, ask. If you aren't comfortable with the answers, don't participate in the project.

Choosing to Manage Your Own Care

As we have discussed, some people are choosing DNA-related testing that avoids traditional doctors and insurers entirely. These direct-to consumer routes usually involve Web-based companies that offer genetic testing on demand, and return results directly to you. The practice has proven popular among some consumers and advocacy groups for people with genetic conditions. They see direct-to-consumer testing as a way for people to take control of their gene information without uncomfortable questions from doctors or insurers.

Some genomic specialists and medical privacy experts warn against direct-to-consumer testing, saying those who choose this option may face a unique set of concerns. Because HIPAA applies primarily to health care providers, and some genetic testing firms may not be legally defined as a health care provider, federal medical privacy laws may not always cover genetic information and testing firms. Some of these companies may collect genetic information and store it indefinitely. Some such firms issue their own privacy policies. Others explicitly state that your DNA information will be passed on to public or private research projects.

If you are considering a direct-to-consumer genetic test, genetic experts advise the following cautions when it comes to your privacy and the use of your DNA information:

- Review the company's privacy and security policies carefully.
- If a company makes no mention of HIPAA, GINA, or medical privacy, ask why. The firm may consider itself exempt.
- Find out how the company protects customer information from electronic theft, and ask if any such information has been stolen or shared in the past.
- Ask if the firm shares patient information or DNA with outside medical researchers or companies, or if it uses your information for its own research purposes.
- Ask about consumer complaints. You can also check with state

RED FLAG!

Some Important Terms You'll Find on Genetic Testing Web Sites

When you visit the Web site of a direct-to-consumer genetic testing company, you'll see many terms that appear to relate to your privacy. Here's what three of them do— and don't—mean:

- **Security.** This term usually applies to your electronic communications with the company and how those communications are shielded from outside viewers. A secure site, for example, usually carries electronic protections that block others from reading your communications with the company. This is an important safeguard if you're discussing your health concerns with the company by email or receiving test results online.
- **Personal information.** This term usually applies to information that reveals your identity, such as your name, address, and billing information. Some companies have policies that clearly spell out when they'll ask for your personal information, and how that information might be attached to any genetic records you have with the company. Others do not have a clear policy. If a company doesn't, ask for details.
- **Personal health information.** This term applies to any of your health information connected to the company. It could mean details of your medical history that you choose to share with the company. It could also include genetic test results. Some companies offer clear policies for how and when they'll view, share, and use your personal health or genetic information. Others may not, so if you feel unsure about how your health information may be handled, ask for specifics or consider taking your business elsewhere.

regulators, such as those that handle consumer complaints, in the state where the company is licensed to do business.

- While some firms advertise that they are CLIA-certified, keep in mind that such certification says nothing about the firm's privacy protections. CLIA certification only means that labs affiliated with the company operate according to federal science standards.

If You've Already Been Diagnosed with a Genetic Illness

People with serious genetic diseases, such as the neurological disorder Huntington's disease, face the same challenges as any person with a major illness. Under HIPAA, they cannot be excluded from most group health plans. But they have been denied individual insurance coverage, according to patient support groups. Huntington's patients have also reported trouble landing jobs at firms that conduct pre-employment medical tests, saying the employers do not want the expense of insuring them.

If you've been diagnosed with a genetic illness, here are some steps you can take to help protect your insurance coverage:

- Contact the Medical Information Bureau to see if you have a file with the group. If so, request a copy. You'll find more information on how to do that earlier in this chapter.
- Opt for group health insurance whenever possible, which gives you more protection from unfavorable insurance decisions.
- Read the fine print in your insurer's policies on your condition. Coverage options vary from company to company.
- Talk to your genetic counselor, as well as others with your condition. Counselors have often helped other patients with insurance problems and may know additional resources you can pursue. Other patients will also have valuable experience to share.

Special Considerations for Ethnic Minorities

Many ethnic minorities say they feel especially vulnerable to genetic discrimination. For some recent immigrants with limited English skills, information on genetic care and privacy may not be easily available in their native language. Many minorities, who often lack good health insurance, also have less access to specialists in any area of medicine, including genomics. And some groups are suspicious of genomic programs, believing their use may mean further discrimination.

Those fears, unfortunately, reflect memories from an earlier era. In the early 1970s, a well-intentioned public health campaign driven by doctors and some black civil rights leaders led to a broad federal and state-based effort to provide better testing and care for sickle cell anemia. The condition affects African-Americans more often than any other group in the United States, and community leaders charged the health of black sickle cell patients had been neglected for too long. The initiative aimed to improve everything from carrier testing to newborn screening and patient care.

But different states started offering their own versions of the program, sometimes in ways that stigmatized people with the sickle cell gene. Between 1970 and 1972, twelve states and the District of Columbia passed laws requiring mandatory sickle cell testing for African-Americans. The results of those tests were often interpreted incorrectly, equating non-symptomatic carriers of sickle cell trait with patients who had sickle cell disease.

With few protections against genetic discrimination in place at the time, blacks who tested positive for sickle cell trait began to find themselves denied jobs and insurance. New York State required sickle cell testing for all marriage license applicants "not of the Caucasian, Indian, or Oriental races." Washington, D.C.'s law mistakenly implied that sickle cell disease was a communicable illness easily passed from person to person, much like a cold or the flu, raising the threat of confinement or isolation. Not surprisingly, some African-Americans began to view the improved sickle cell care as little more than an organized discrimination campaign that threatened their families and livelihoods.

More knowledgeable doctors and policy makers, seeing their efforts to improve sickle cell care backfire, scrambled to put better programs in place. In 1972, the passage of the National Sickle Cell Anemia Control Act set new standards for sickle cell testing and care that eliminated many of the earlier problems. In the meantime, however, the public's trust had been badly damaged. Genetic counselors and other experts suggest that concerned members of minority communities ask the following questions when considering genomic care:

- If you or members of your family are not proficient in English, are informational materials available in your native language? If not, many large health care centers offer translators for medical care, including genetic counseling sessions.
- If you are considering genetic testing, ask about the test's track record in your community. Some tests, such as cystic fibrosis or sickle cell tests, are designed to detect disease-causing mutations most common to a particular ethnic group, but they may miss less common mutations found in different ethnic groups.

If You Are a Federal Employee

When it comes to protection from genetic bias on the job, people who work for the many branches of the federal government encounter different laws. One group of government workers—federal civilian employees—has its own set of protections. But members of the military routinely face genetic testing and gene-based decisions, and are not covered by GINA or similar laws.

In February 2000, president Bill Clinton signed an executive order banning every federal department and agency from using genetic information in any hiring or promotion action affecting civilian employees. By using an executive order, Clinton was able to circumvent Congress, where similar reforms for all Americans had been blocked.

The executive order prohibits federal employers from:

- Requiring or requesting genetic tests as a condition of being hired, receiving benefits, or evaluating a civilian worker's ability to perform a job.
- Using protected genetic information to classify civilian employees in a manner that deprives them of promotions or transfers.
- Obtaining or disclosing genetic information about civilian employees or potential employees, except when it is necessary to provide medical treatment to employees, ensure workplace health and safety, or provide occupational and health researchers access to data.

But Clinton's order didn't cover one large sector of people working in public service—members of the military. Nor does GINA. The U.S. military routinely takes DNA samples from its members and uses their information to help make work assignments, fire or promote someone, and determine health care benefits. Military leaders say the information is necessary to make sure military personnel receive the right health care and work placements.

The use of this genetic information by the military has been mixed. Previously, some members of the military say that their genetic information was used as grounds for dismissal or to cut off their health and disability benefits. Some former members of the military have said their genetic illnesses were termed pre-existing conditions, and used as grounds for cutting off health care services or disability payments. More recently, however, a new policy states that service members may be medically

Did You Know ?

Despite the firm rules of the U.S. military's genetic testing policy, some service members have been able win legal challenges to some parts of the program:

- In the late 1990s, a 15-year veteran of the U.S. Marine Corps who developed genetically linked cancer during his years of service successfully fought a decision to dismiss him from the military without any health or disability benefits. An appeals board reversed an early ruling and awarded the Marine full retirement with medical benefits.
- In the mid-1990s, two Marines refused orders to give DNA samples before being deployed for duty. The two said they were not comfortable with how their samples might be stored or used. The Marines faced court martial for violating orders. In 1996, a military judge ordered only light punishment for the two Marines and said they did not have to give DNA samples. The judge's order also allowed the Marines to leave the service with an honorable discharge.

retired with benefits if, after six months, their disability was not noted at the time they joined the service.

If you are a member of the military who has lost rank, status, or benefits because of a genetic condition, or been expelled from the service, experts recommend pursuing an appeal. Some former service members have had their rank or benefits restored after filing appeals. For more information, contact The Genetics and Public Policy Center at Johns Hopkins University (www.dnapolicy.org). The center has conducted research and public discussions on the use of genomic information in the military.

FREQUENTLY ASKED QUESTIONS ON GENOMIC PRIVACY

Q. Every doctor's office I visit gives me some disclosure of information form to fill out. How does this relate to my genomic information?

A. HIPAA regulations require that health care providers give you these forms to read and sign. These disclosure forms cover all your medical information, including your genomic information. Your doctor's office cannot share your medical information, including your genomic information, with other caregivers or your insurance company, if you haven't signed a disclosure form. Read disclosure forms carefully before you sign them. You can also try deleting some sections of the form you find unacceptable, although some medical institutions do not allow this. If you don't understand parts of the form, ask to speak to a privacy specialist who works with your doctor's office.

Q. I'd like to try a direct-to-consumer genetic test I saw online. The testing company's Web site says my results will be sent directly to me and treated confidentially. Isn't that enough reassurance?

A. No. A vague promise of confidentiality is not the same as a legally binding guarantee. That promise, for example, may only cover the instance in which your test results are sent to you. It says nothing about how your test results may be later released to others. See if the company is HIPAA-compliant, or if it has a separate privacy policy. The firm should also have a terms-and-conditions agreement that outlines how your DNA information will be handled and used. Read any such documents carefully. If the firm doesn't comply with HIPAA or offer a thorough privacy policy or terms and conditions agreement, consider taking your business elsewhere.

Q. My doctor's office is urging me to donate some DNA to a gene bank. My doctor's office is covered by HIPAA. Doesn't that mean my donation is protected, too?

A. No. The gene bank is probably separate from your doctor's office, and gene banks or research experiments often aren't covered by HIPAA or other federal privacy rules. To understand how the gene bank will protect your identity and use your DNA, read its privacy and use policies, and see how the gene bank's scientists plan to comply with confidentiality rules established by scientific oversight boards. These privacy standards may not be the same as your doctor's.

KEEP IN MIND

As your health care becomes more personalized, these key points can help you protect your privacy and shield you from potential discrimination.

The Genetic Information Nondiscrimination Act (GINA) was passed in 2008 and implemented in 2009. This federal law provides protection for genomic information in health insurance and employment situations. Other forms of health-related insurance, such as disability or life insurance, however, are not covered by the law. While GINA serves as a baseline for protection, some states have also passed strong laws of their own. See the resources listed earlier in this chapter to start learning more about the laws in your state.

In general, you receive better privacy protection when you receive care from established, traditional medical networks. In other gene-related realms, such as direct-to-consumer genetic testing or research projects, you may receive less protection, as the same federal laws may not apply.

Don't assume that direct-to-consumer genetic testing companies automatically protect your privacy. Review whatever privacy policies and terms-and-conditions agreements they offer and ask detailed questions before using their services.

Gene experts hope that as genomic health care becomes more and more a part of everyday health care, the laws that protect your privacy and control the use of your genomic information will continue to improve. These shifting rules are just one part of the rapidly changing world of genomics, where new advances arrive every day. Next, we look at some of the big discoveries poised to further reshape your personalized medicine health kit.

CHAPTER NINE

YOUR GENES AND YOUR HEALTH: WHAT LIES AHEAD

Mark Origer, battling a deadly type of skin cancer, never expected to live long enough to walk his daughter down the aisle at her wedding. Yet there he was, in a dark suit with a rose pinned to his lapel, proudly escorting Katie in her flowing white dress.

The family scene that autumn day—a proud father with a beautiful daughter on his arm—plays out across the country countless times each year. But the breakthrough that let Origer share that experience was anything but common. In 2004, almost a year before Katie's wedding, Origer had slid into the last stages of malignant melanoma. About 8,000 Americans die every year from this cancer, which can spread throughout the body, turning up in a new spot after doctors think they've controlled it in another. With nowhere else to turn, Origer took one last chance.

The Wisconsin man joined an experiment in which scientists would remove some of his body's disease-fighting cells, filling them with new genes skilled at finding and destroying cancer. The scientists would then inject the supercharged cells back into Origer's blood. Going in, the prospects didn't look good. Many efforts in this realm of experimental treatment, known as gene therapy, had failed before. But Origer had nothing left to lose.

A month later, Origer's doctors gave him a cancer check-up, and astonished smiles spread across their faces. His tumors had started to shrink. By the time of Katie's wedding, only one tumor lingered in Origer's body, small enough for surgeons to remove. Two years after receiving his gene therapy, Origer remained cancer-free.

"I know how fortunate I am," Origer said when the news of his cancer recovery was announced. "Not everybody is that lucky."

Few genomic scientists start medical experiments expecting that they'll allow a dying man to plan his daughter's wedding instead of his own funeral. But Origer's personal reversal of fortune signals an important victory in one of the biggest medical research efforts of our time. All around the world, thousands of scientists are trying to push genomic medicine to the next level by altering the DNA behind disease. In this chapter, we look at some of the most interesting and promising genomic advances being developed to improve your health.

Using the tools of genetic engineering—powerful supercomputers and laboratory techniques that let them copy, alter, and move genes—these researchers are transforming science into new types of gene-centered medicine. Some seek to repair risk-related DNA or silence genes that cause illness. Others push the boundaries of genomic care further, inserting new genes into the body as part of gene therapy experiments. Some even remove a special type of highly versatile cells—known as stem

RED FLAG!

Joining a Genomic Experiment: Questions to Ask

Whether you simply hope to help the cause of genomic science or want to try new treatments for a serious health problem, there are usually plenty of ongoing research projects looking for volunteers. Hundreds of gene-related clinical trials operate in the United States at any given time, and one or more of them may be looking for trial participants just like you.

Before you rush to sign up, there are some important points to consider, especially if you join a trial that is testing a new treatment. Remember that these trials are experiments with no guarantees. The new treatment may not work for you. It may carry serious or even life-threatening side effects. And it may require a significant amount of your time and attention, including trips to the center where the trial is based, hospital stays, and follow-up visits with the research team.

Whether the trial tests a new treatment or not, reputable scientific studies all follow some basic rules to protect your privacy and well-being. Ask the following questions of any clinical trial you might join:

- Does the trial operate under a set of guidelines called a research protocol?
- Is this protocol available for your review, and does the trial offer staff members who can help explain it to you?
- What kind of tests and experimental treatments are involved?
- Have these procedures been tested before, and why does the trial team think they might be effective?
- How will the trial affect my daily life?
- Who will pay the costs of the trial, including any experimental treatment?
- Who will be in charge of my care? Will my regular doctor be involved?
- Will I be informed of the results of the trial?
- Does the trial include any follow-up care?

The National Institutes of Health offers a good place to start looking for clinical trials operating under established scientific guidelines. Visit the Web site www.clinicaltrials.gov to find a searchable database of clinical trials by type and location. The site also offers a great overview of the entire clinical trial process. It's worth learning about how trials work, because the knowledge will help you make faster, more informed decisions should you ever find you'd like to participate.

cells—from the tissues of grown adults or human embryos, in the hopes of coaxing them into providing cures for disease or new tissues for people with injuries.

If you think this work seems packed with big doses of excitement and concern, you'd be right on both counts. Many areas of genomic research represent some of the most important science of our time, but they are also some of the most uncertain—and controversial. For example, the gene therapy experiment that Mark Origer took part in included 17 melanoma patients. Only two, Origer and one other man, maintained high levels of the gene therapy treatment in their blood and saw substantial improvement. Scientists who led the project couldn't identify why. Many other gene therapy efforts have failed, and in a few, a handful of patients have died or developed cancer after receiving their experimental treatment. The harvesting and use of cells from human embryos, known as embryonic stem cell research, presents one of the most significant scientific controversies we face as a society.

As a result, leaders in genomic research never claim that their work is anything close to a quick guarantee of healing. Emerging areas of genomic medicine remain an evolving, inexact science. Our bodies carry

Genomic Research: A Long Process

Why does it usually take years, even decades, to develop medical treatments from new sciences such as genomic research? The answer lies in the deliberate steps scientists take to ensure that their work doesn't do more harm than good.

Many gene research experiments, for example, start by testing gene manipulations or medicines on human or animal cells grown in labs. Experiments can be conducted on these cells without harming a living creature. After cell studies, many scientists then move on to testing treatments in mice or other animals. Only if cell and animal studies show promise do most scientists even begin considering human medical experiments. Once they do, they must test their new treatment in three phases—a small study that evaluates the treatment's safety, a larger one that establishes its effectiveness, and an even broader one that confirms its effectiveness and watches for side effects. New treatments must succeed in all three phases to be approved for use.

The need to fulfill all these steps explains why a promising piece of gene research news may not lead to new treatments for many years. Scientists studying the autism-related condition Rett syndrome, for example, recently announced the exciting news that they had reversed the condition in a group of mice. These mice had been genetically engineered to carry the gene mutation that causes Rett syndrome, and the research team was able to counteract the mutation and reverse the mice's symptoms. Families of children with Rett syndrome gladly greeted the news as a major breakthrough. But given all the steps these scientists must now follow to see if their work can yield a treatment for people, it will probably be years before the work with Rett mice means help for children with the condition.

strong defenses to protect our genes from change and tampering—including the tinkering of doctors and scientists. Many of these advances are being scrutinized carefully by ethicists and lawmakers. Still, if genomic scientists' theories prove right, one of these new ways of working with your genome might just give you the gift Mark Origer received—a new chance at a healthier life.

We'll start with a look at one of the most powerful tools genomic science is developing to protect your health—detecting and identifying the DNA of harmful microscopic invaders.

DETECTING DANGEROUS DNA

Every time you catch the flu, the germs that make you sick invade your body with their own genetic code. If you come down with an illness that doctors haven't seen before, isolating and reading this genetic information can reveal exactly what you've got, and how to fight it. Scientists are quickly learning how to spot the genetic signatures of disease-causing intruders, such as germs or cancer cells, in a person's blood or tissues, and then use that information to limit the harm they cause.

In recent years, genomic science has scored some impressive victories against invasive diseases by learning how to pinpoint their DNA:

- **Rapid identification of new diseases.** When a deadly new virus called SARS (severe acute respiratory syndrome) began sickening thousands of people around the world in 2003, doctors confronting the unfamiliar pathogen weren't sure how to treat or stop it. They sent samples of the virus to teams of genomic detectives around the world, who sprang into action. Picking apart the genes of the SARS virus, researchers in the United States and Canada sequenced all of its DNA within days. The information revealed that SARS is related to a familiar group of respiratory viruses, giving doctors better ways to detect SARS and treat it. It's also proven essential to ongoing efforts to develop a SARS vaccine.

Did You Know ?

In the mid-1980s, multiple teams of researchers needed more than two years to identify the human immunodeficiency virus (HIV) as the cause of AIDS (acquired immunodeficiency syndrome) and sequence HIV's DNA. In 2004, researchers took about 24 hours to establish that SARS belongs to a familiar family of respiratory viruses, and about another four days to sequence the DNA of the two major SARS strains. This difference reflects, in part, just how much genomic tools have improved over the years—and how much these improvements strengthen our hand against new diseases.

- **Detecting infections earlier.** Women who contract sexually transmitted diseases such as the human papillomavirus (HPV), gonorrhea, or chlamydia often aren't aware of these silent infections until they have left substantial physical damage. HPV, for example, is closely linked to cervical cancer, and long-term chlamydia infection leaves some women infertile. Traditional tests for these diseases haven't always proven reliable at finding them early. But new gene-based tests can catch these invaders before they cause serious symptoms by detecting their DNA. A gene test that looks for the genetic signatures of certain strains of HPV, for example, is gradually replacing the traditional Pap smear as the standard way of assessing a woman's risk of cervical cancer. A similar gene test can detect gonorrhea or chlamydia infection.

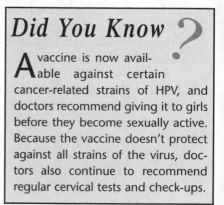

Did You Know ?

A vaccine is now available against certain cancer-related strains of HPV, and doctors recommend giving it to girls before they become sexually active. Because the vaccine doesn't protect against all strains of the virus, doctors also continue to recommend regular cervical tests and check-ups.

- **Detecting cancer earlier.** Thanks to improved understanding of cancer-causing genes and how they work, scientists now know that cancerous cells leave telltale traces of their presence in a person's blood long before they cause a noticeable lump or other symptoms. Cancerous cells, due to certain instructions carried in their genes, express unique types and levels of certain proteins. If you can find even small amounts of these proteins, scientists say, you know cancer is at work. Cancer researchers are now working to develop reliable blood tests that detect these proteins, in the hopes of catching cancer at its earliest stages. So far, the accuracy of these tests varies, but their overall quality is improving. In one such experiment involving breast cancer, for example, a blood test for certain cancer-related proteins accurately detected cancer in more than 90 percent of cases. (For another example, a new saliva test for oral cancer, see Chapter 5.)

The ability to detect and locate genetic material from risky cells or microbes, however, can't begin to address all the intricacies of DNA. To do that, other scientists are looking beyond DNA, focusing on the infrastructure that helps it function.

Revealing the Epigenome

While your genes carry the codes for your body's building blocks, they don't work alone. Your genome is intertwined with another vital set of biological instructions, your epigenome. The term, which literally means "on the genome," refers to an elaborate web of biochemical compounds that works closely with your genome to regulate its function. The cells of your skin, hair, and eyes, for example, all have the same DNA. But each of these features looks quite distinct, thanks to epigenetic influences that determine which segments of your DNA are at work in different parts of your body.

As scientific understanding of the epigenome improves, it is becoming clear that your epigenome does more than make your skin cells different from your hair cells. Your epigenome can change according to your environment. That means it also affects the function of DNA related to your health. And like your genes, your epigenome can become damaged by toxins and other harmful substances. In many types of cancer, for example, scientists have found epigenetic changes alongside cancerous DNA mutations. Some now theorize that many cancers are caused by this mix of DNA and epigenetic damage. Like your DNA, the features of your epigenome can also be passed from one generation to the next, making epigenetics a growing focus of research into how illnesses are inherited.

If that makes the epigenome sound like just one more health headache, it's important to note that epigenetics also offers promising avenues for improving health. Studies show that your epigenome may sometimes be more receptive to therapies than your DNA, responding well to good basic preventive health measures and treatments that influence how different genes are expressed. While this research is still in its early stages, scientists have made progress using epigenetic therapy against a few diseases, especially some forms of cancer.

To see epigenetics in action, we next discuss a technique called RNAi, which aims to put risk-related DNA on mute.

SILENCING RISK-RELATED GENES

What if risk-related DNA could be stopped from harming your health without repairing or replacing it? What if there was some way to muffle it, stopping it from issuing instructions that might make you sick?

That's the goal of an emerging genomic technology working to silence risk-related DNA. Called RNA interference, or RNAi, this technique focuses on blocking harmful DNA's ability to do its work. As you may remember from Chapter 1, RNA is a close cousin of DNA, helping DNA copy itself and issue instructions for making proteins. If you can block the RNA helping a particular piece of DNA to release its protein instructions, you've effectively cut off that DNA's ability to do its job. Through such interference with the RNA connected to certain disease-linked genes and DNA, scientists are seeing whether they can halt or cure a wide range of health problems.

An early focus of human RNAi trials has been a disease called macular degeneration, a leading cause of blindness that affects more than one million older Americans. One major form of macular degeneration is triggered by too much of a protein called VEGF, which fuels blood vessel growth. Too much VEGF in your body can create too many blood vessels near your retina, a tissue that forms a vital part of your vision. Over time, these extra blood vessels in the retina leak, obscuring and sometimes even

A Speedy Prize for RNAi

For most researchers who win science's top prize, a Nobel award doesn't arrive for decades. The scientific community usually wants to see how a discovery unfolds over time before conferring its top honor. So when two American scientists received a 2006 Nobel Prize in medicine for breakthrough findings on RNAi that they'd announced only eight years before, the entire gene research world paid attention. Andrew Fire and Craig Mello's Nobel award for research they published in 1998, describing how to silence RNA from a specific gene, shows the widespread belief that RNAi will deliver big health benefits to many people soon.

destroying a person's eyesight. So far, tests of RNAi drugs to silence the VEGF gene have shown promising results in stopping, and sometimes even reversing, vision loss in macular degeneration. RNAi experiments are also underway against a wide variety of other health problems, including HIV, high cholesterol, cancer, and the currently incurable neurological disorder Huntington's disease.

While early successes in RNAi experiments have been promising, scientists still face serious obstacles in making RNAi a regular part of medical care. RNAi therapies need to reach their targets quickly to be effective, and scientists have found it challenging to give people doses that last long enough to help. RNAi drugs for macular degeneration, for example, have a good chance of working because they can be injected straight into the eye. Reaching deeper tissues that need treatment, however, remains a challenge. It's also not always easy to ensure that an RNAi treatment only disrupts the RNA it is intended to target. Many different versions of RNA are structurally similar, and an imprecise RNA therapy could disrupt healthy genes as well as risk-related ones. Scientists estimate that RNAi's overall risk for such straying off-target at about 10 percent.

Despite these obstacles, many scientists remain optimistic about the health benefits to be gained from RNAi. A large number of RNAi treatments are either being studied or should start clinical trials within the next five years.

SIZING UP YOUR GENOME'S SAFETY STRAPS

Alongside your genes, the biological packaging that protects your personal genome also has something important to say about your health. Scientists are learning that telomeres, tiny bits of DNA that help hold the pieces of your genome together, have connections to health concerns such as aging, cancer, and heart disease. Telomeres don't carry any genetic operating instructions that might influence these conditions, but they do help preserve the health and structure of your genes. So, if telomeres erode, that may affect how well some aspects of your body functions.

To understand how telomeres keep your DNA healthy, think back to how your genome is formed. As you may remember from the overview of your genome in Chapter 1, your genes and supporting DNA string together to form chromosomes. You have 46 of them, each held together at the ends by telomeres. These safety straps are made up of stretches of DNA, and they help keep your chromosomes from fraying, especially when your chromosomes divide and copy themselves to make DNA for new cells in your body. That's because copying chromosomes requires a sacrifice. For complex biological reasons, every division and copying of your chromosomes leaves a few base letters off the ends. If those bases went missing from a functional gene, that gene might stop working normally, and your health could suffer. So telomeres, standing guard at the ends of your chromosomes, give up a few of their bases instead. They shed bases during chromosome copying so that your genes stay intact.

Over time, though, all this sacrifice takes a toll on your telomeres. Telomeres get some help replacing lost bases from a substance in your body called telomerase, but as you age, your available amounts of telomerase start to run thin. Over time, the loss of bases with each cell division leaves telomeres with few extras to spare, making your chromosomes more vulnerable. Cells that divide often, such as your blood cells, suffer most. When most people are young, for example, the telomeres in the chromosomes of their blood cells contain anywhere from 10,000 to 20,000 bases. In older people, by contrast, such telomeres usually have only a few thousand bases.

By measuring the length of people's telomeres, scientists have since linked these tiny DNA safety straps to a number of different conditions:

- **Aging.** According to some gene research, shorter telomeres may equal a shorter life. One group of scientists, for example, found that people over the age of 60 with shorter telomeres were more at risk of death from both heart disease and infectious illnesses than were similarly aged people with longer telomeres.

Easy Clues to Telomeres

The first clues to the importance of telomeres came from people with an extremely rare genetic illness that reduces their amount of telomerase and leads to abnormally short telomeres at a young age. People with this condition, called dyskeratosis congenita, suffer abrupt premature aging and often die in their teens from bone marrow failure, serious internal infections, or cancer. The condition affects only about 1 in 1 million people. But in the 1980s and 1990s, as scientists realized the disorder was caused by genes that affect telomeres and telomerase, they also started linking telomeres to more common health conditions.

Research Studies Offer Both Hope and Frustration

Dave (whom you met in Chapter 7) was an executive because he was a good researcher—he could uncover financial problems in companies when no one else could. So when his mother was diagnosed with Alzheimer's disease, he began researching and learned of a new drug that was being used for mildly affected Alzheimer's disease patients in a phase III study. A phase III study, he read, is when an experimental drug is given to between 1,000 and 3,000 people to make sure it works, to discover side effects, and to collect information that will allow the drug to be used safely. In the phase II study, this drug had shown promise of stopping or even reversing signs of Alzheimer's disease. Dave hoped this drug could improve his mother's ability to handle daily household activities enough so she could cook without him worrying that she had left the burners on.

Because of the voluntary nature of research, Dave's mother would not be allowed to enroll unless she clearly understood the purpose and process of the research. Dave was concerned about this aspect because there were days when her cognitive abilities were limited. The first explanation took quite a while, and the coordinator would not let her start until after a week had passed and she was still able to answer questions about the study. Dave was pleased when she seemed to understand relatively well and still wanted to join. And as her caretaker, Dave also had to enroll, because he would be participating as well, reporting how the drug impacted her daily functioning.

Then Dave found out that study participants would be "randomized," meaning they would not be told whether they were receiving the drug being tested or a placebo. If his mom was going to be in a study, he really wanted her to get the drug that would help! It was explained to him there would have been bias in the study if anything other than a computer assigned which participants should receive the drug. And, doctors pointed out, sometimes new drugs don't work or can even cause harm—the purpose of this phase III trial was to see if the drug would help, because they didn't know for sure that it would. On the other hand, regardless of whether she got the experimental drug or the placebo, as part of the study, she would receive regular check-ups by knowledgeable people in the field, an aspect that was reassuring to Dave.

After his mom had been in the trial for a while, Dave got to thinking. If this drug could stop or possibly improve symptoms for people with mild Alzheimer's disease, could it possibly benefit people *before* the disease even starts?

So Dave asked me about that type of study, because he wanted to be in it—now! To his disappointment, it would be several years before such a study would be launched. Additionally, the study would probably begin with people at highest risk, so to join, he would have to decide if he wanted to know his *ApoE* e4 mutation status after all. But long before such a study could take place, researchers needed to know that the drug helped people with the disease for more than a few years, and they needed to carefully examine the drug's side effects. It is one thing to give a drug with side effects to a person who is sick, but the rules are stricter when giving a drug to a person who is well. We both hoped that the drug would help his mother and that in the future, a trial would be available for him as well.

Bottom line: As a genetic counselor who has worked with many rare conditions, I understand the incredibly important role of research. I also understand the frustrations people have when they are faced with the opportunity to be in a research study. But it is only in the powerful partnership of scientists, clinicians, and patients that clinical research trials can happen and the knowledge shared in this book can exist. I so appreciate all the individuals who have made the difficult decision to participate in research—it isn't easy, but without you, discoveries would not happen.

- **Cancer.** Cells with shortened telomeres may be a factor in both the cause and progress of some cancers. Scientists have found cells with unusually short telomeres in many different types of cancer, including bone, kidney, and prostate malignancies.
- **Heart disease.** Some researchers have found that men with shorter telomeres in their white blood cells are about twice as likely to develop coronary artery disease. When some of these men were treated with a common cholesterol-lowering drug called a statin, however, this increased risk largely disappeared.

Big questions surround these interesting connections between telomeres, aging, and illness. Do shorter telomeres trigger decline or sickness? Or are they just a sign of aging or illness, much in the way that grey hair is only an indicator of advancing years, not a cause. Do short telomeres cause cancer, or do they simply reflect that cancerous cells divide quickly and may burn through telomeres at a rapid clip? Research in other areas of aging shows that telomeres can't be the only factor in the physical decline that comes with time. And telomere lengths vary widely from person to person at birth. What exactly is a healthy amount of telomeres? Are different numbers of telomeres normal for different population groups?

Until scientists can answer such questions, it will be difficult to develop medical tests that measure telomeres in useful ways. As research progresses, however, you can expect a steady flow of interesting news on how these chromosomal safety straps affect the health of your genes and your body.

Counting Out Your DNA

The story of your genome is told not only in letters, but also in numbers.

Your DNA is made up of billions of bases, or the letters that spell out genetic code. As we mentioned at the start of this book, some of these letters read differently from person to person—you may have an A in one spot, while the person sitting next to you at work has a T in the same place. But these differences can also come in terms of quantity. At a different place on your genome, for example, you may have a G. The person sitting next to you at work may also have a G at that spot, or GGG, or no base at that point at all.

These differences in quantities of genetic material are called copy number variants or repeats. In a very limited way, scientists have understood the importance of differences in DNA numbers for decades. For example, two of the disorders discussed in Chapter 7, Huntington disease and Fragile X syndrome, are triggered by different series of bases that repeat themselves too many times. Down syndrome arises when three copies of a chromosome are present, instead of the regular two.

Now, recent research shows that numerous copy number variants are common from person to person, and likely have important implications for health. Some copy number variants on certain spots on the human genome, for example, have been linked to heart disease, cataracts, or schizophrenia.

Scientists say they still have a lot to learn about copy number variants, and they are working to create an easy, affordable way to both spell out and count out most people's DNA. But as research into copy number variants progresses, you can expect to hear more about telling your DNA's story by its numbers.

REPAIRING YOUR GENOME

If one of your genes had a risk-related variant, imagine being able to do more than just find ways to live with that reality. Imagine that your doctor could somehow counteract or alter your genome, fixing the error and allowing your body to operate more smoothly.

This field of gene discovery, known as gene therapy, represents one of the most hopeful goals of genomic medicine. It's also perhaps the most difficult. Your body cloaks your genome with sophisticated layers of protection that are extremely difficult to penetrate. These safeguards are essential for keeping your genes healthy, but they also make reaching a faulty gene and fixing it a major challenge. Any actual fixes to genes require entering the cell walls that protect them—something that's difficult to do without destroying the cell entirely. And since just about every cell in your body contains a full copy of your genome, gene fixes would have to enter thousands or millions of cells at once for the repair to have any meaningful effect.

These challenges have kept attempts at true gene repair in a stop-start pattern for more than a decade, with limited success. The first human experiments with gene therapy started in 1990, and for a time focused on genetically altered viruses that might deliver healthy versions of human genes straight into cells. This area of research suffered a setback, however, when a teenage boy with an inherited metabolic disorder died after receiving an experimental virus-delivered gene therapy treatment. Doctors later linked his death to a severe reaction to the virus. Further setbacks in viral gene therapy experiments, involving children in a French gene therapy study who developed leukemia, led U.S. health officials to reconsider such research until risks can be reduced.

Currently, the vast majority of gene therapy protocols involve various cancers, where the target is a somatic cell. However, gene therapy studies are being conducted for other conditions, such as

Did You Know ?

Despite all the setbacks gene therapy research has suffered, the field remains one of high interest to people with serious or incurable genetic illness, who know that science offers their best prospect for a turnaround. According to one scientific estimate, more than 3,000 people have participated in gene therapy experiments—a sign of the hope patients have in this research and the scientists leading it.

severe combined immunodeficiency, one of the first conditions to benefit from gene therapy trials. A list of active trials, which continuously changes, can be found at www.clinicaltrials.gov.

In the meantime, scientists have focused on a less ambitious, but also less risky, form of gene therapy. These experiments rely on putting genetically healthy versions of cells into the bodies of people with risk-related genes, in the hopes that the healthy cells will counteract the defective ones. It's this approach that led to Mark Origer's recent cancer recovery. In the experiment he joined, scientists took disease-fighting blood cells from 17 people with melanoma, genetically rebuilding the cells as better cancer fighters. Then they injected the cells back into the patients. The results were modest in number, but promising in their potential. Two of the 17 saw their cancer virtually disappear. And in a happy shift from some uses of virus-based gene therapy, none of the patients got sick from their re-engineered blood cells.

In practical terms, though, gene therapy still faces big questions and obstacles. In Origer's experiment, for example, 15 patients didn't sustain high enough levels of the new cells to help beat back their cancer. Scientists still have to answer many questions about why gene therapy has so far proven erratic or ineffective in so many different cases. But with a wide variety of gene therapy experiments underway, it's likely that researchers will make steady progress on tackling these problems.

COPYING GENES, COPYING GENOMES

Sometimes scientists try to work beyond gene repair. Instead, they try to copy genes—sometimes just a few, sometimes an entire genome's worth—to see if these copies hold medical promise.

This process of copying genes and the life they support is called cloning, and it has become one of the most morally loaded words in all of genomics. Scientists already have the ability to copy individual genes, and sometimes make genomic copies of entire plants or animals. These cloning accomplishments raise the prospect of making genomic copies of humans, an idea that most people say takes the power of gene science too far.

Cloning comes in three main forms:

- DNA cloning, in which individual genes or bits of DNA are copied by merging them with special types of fast-replicating DNA from bacteria. This process is now widely used in science, often to make multiple copies of a particular gene so that it can be analyzed more easily. If a person has a rare disease-causing mutation, for example, a single copy of that mutation can be replicated many times over using this technology, providing plenty of copies for teams of scientists to study.
- Therapeutic cloning, in which a special type of versatile human cell, called a stem cell, is harvested and replicated to see whether it might yield treatments for diseases such as spinal cord injuries,

diabetes, or Parkinson's disease. Stem cells can be taken from either adult tissues or human embryos. Embryonic stem cells are the more flexible kind, able to grow into many different types of tissue. But harvesting these stem cells requires destroying the embryos that form them, making this form of stem cell research one of the most controversial issues in contemporary science. People hoping for therapies derived from stem cell research say that developing help for ailing people should be the top priority. Others counter that destroying any human life, even one just a few cells in size, is wrong and should be illegal.

• Reproductive cloning, in which entire creatures are copied by inserting a full version of their genome into an egg that has been artificially emptied of its own genes. That egg, now carrying a full genome in the same way that a naturally fertilized one would, may go on to develop normally and produce an infant that is a genetic copy of the creature that provided its genome. This process has been widely tried with animals, and has sometimes produced healthy lambs (including the world-famous cloned sheep "Dolly"), kittens, mice, and even endangered species. In humans, however, the idea of reproductive cloning is even more controversial than stem cells. Many countries ban human reproductive cloning, and major medical organizations oppose it as well, saying it oversteps the bounds of our moral authority and scientific ability.

Cloning inspires more controversy and fear than any other aspect of genomics, and given its potential power, the issues surrounding cloning are well worth debating. It's also important, though, to keep the limits of this technology in mind. Reproductive cloning has a dismal success rate. More than 90 percent of cloning attempts in animals fail to produce a healthy baby animal. If they do fully develop and are born, many cloned animals suffer from disease at much higher rates than normal animals, and others die early of mysterious causes.

Right now, the level of controversy around cloning is far larger than its ability to provide any large-scale health benefits. That lag gives us all a valuable gift—time to make decisions about how we want cloning technologies to be used. Many other aspects of genomic science—even something as basic as genetic testing—have gone to work in the world before we've been sure how we want to handle them. In this case, if we talk as a society before we clone, we have time to reach a consensus on what we consider to be ethical uses of this powerful technology.

FREQUENTLY ASKED QUESTIONS ON THE FUTURE OF GENOMIC MEDICINE

Q. When my mom had cancer, we tried enrolling her in an experiment that was testing a new gene therapy. But the people leading the study said her cancer was too advanced, and wouldn't include her. She died a couple of months later. I'm still really angry with the scientists who led that trial. People who want to join these experiments are desperate sometimes. Why are there so many impossible rules about participating?

A. First of all, know that scientists everywhere take your frustration seriously. No one who conducts a medical experiment takes turning people away lightly. But the tough truth about clinical trials, including genomic trials, is that they are experiments, not treatments. Experiments must follow strict rules so that their results have validity. If a new gene therapy is being tested as a way to fight early stage cancer, for example, and the scientists in charge then include people with more advanced cancer, they won't be able to accurately answer the question that launched their experiment. Scientists, therefore, have to stick to the rules of their trial when they sign people up—a fact that produces good research, but also often causes anger and confusion in those who get turned away. And sometimes, people who don't meet the criteria for a trial may still get a break. Some trials operate under expanded access rules that allow additional people to join if they might benefit from the treatment being studied. To find out if a trial offers expanded access, talk to your doctor or the research group running the trial.

Q. *When I hear news about gene experiments, it's usually good, but what happens to people who are part of unsuccessful experiments? They don't seem to make headlines the way the big breakthroughs do.*

A. You're right. News of genomic research usually focuses on the extremes—experiments that produce big discoveries or mistakes. But most of the time, these experiments unfold less dramatically. In research efforts that fail, people who enroll often simply aren't helped by the treatment being studied. If they have a chronic illness, they may continue to have to manage it with existing treatments. If they have a fatal illness, they may die after the experimental therapy didn't work. People who enter clinical trials do so knowing they are taking a chance, and that an experimental treatment can't offer any guarantees.

Q. *If cloning animals fails often, and the clones that are born have so many health problems, why does anyone pursue more cloning at all? To me, cloning animals is one step away from cloning human beings, and it would be better to drop the whole thing.*

A. Animal cloning may not be as controversial as human cloning, but there are plenty of people who agree with you. On one side are scientists who say that cloning animals provides invaluable information about how genes work, and offers a chance to protect endangered species. There are also plenty of businesses that intend to make money off of cloned animals. On the other side are critics who argue that cloning animals is prohibitively expensive at best and cruel and unethical at worst. As with other aspects of cloning, there are few easy answers to this debate. If you'd like to learn more about cloning, see the Resources section at the end of this book.

Q. I look at where we are with gene research, and I feel like we're living in a time of miracles we don't appreciate. Every breakthrough—even just a new idea—gets hit with a bunch of doomsday critics who say we're marching towards some kind of genetically engineered nightmare. It drives me crazy because I think we're really lucky. The human genome was mapped in our lifetime, and now it's actually helping people. Why is there so much griping about something with this much power?

A. That last word in your question—power—provides all the explanation you seek. We certainly do live in a time of fascinating and important scientific breakthroughs that not only answer big questions about who we are, but have the potential to make major improvements in human health. But that ability to do good also carries the potential for harm. Science and medicine are like any human endeavors, rife with intrigue, suspicion, selfishness, and even greed. Genomic research offers vast benefits, but concerns about the downsides are also vital to its success, steering it to a place where it offers the greatest good.

KEEP IN MIND

Your genes' potential to boost your health doesn't stop with your family history, genetic testing, or even new personalized drugs. Around the world, scientists are working to take genomic care to the next level by analyzing DNA more deeply and learning to work it. Within a few years, you may find that doctors can offer drugs that block instructions issued by risk-related DNA, stopping the harm it does to your body.

Scientists are also studying how structural protections in your DNA affect your health, as well as ways to insert new genes that counteract disease into your body. Some are also seeing if they can manipulate genes in stem cells from human embryos to produce treatments for serious illnesses. These endeavors are medically promising, but they also require many more years of research—and ethical debate—before scientists know if they can be made a routine part of better health.

These experimental developments are well worth watching. But as you finish this book, we also hope you'll take away the knowledge that when it comes to your genes and your health, the future is very much here and now. You don't need to wait for the results of the next big experiment to start making your genes a part of a healthier life. You can start creating your family medical history today, for free, and start seeing what it says about your health. You could undergo genetic testing, much like Kevin Lewis in Chapter 2, and use your results to protect yourself from a family illness. You could look at your family medical history, much like the community of Pima Indians in Chapter 4, and realize that certain foods are better kept out of your kitchen. You could insist on genetic fairness, just like Heidi Williams in Chapter 8, and make use of new laws that help protect you from genetic discrimination. You could take an informed chance, like Mark Origer, and join a genomic experiment that just might help you and others.

You already have the tools to understand your genes more deeply and act on what you find there. You can improve your health, and your family's. Start learning about your own genes. Make choices that make the most of them. Your health now not only reflects how you are, but you can now truly tie it to that most unique part of yourself, the genes that help shape who you are. In making the decision to work with your DNA, you can turn your life—and even your world—into a place where truly personal health can thrive.

Resources

Here is a list of online resources and more information.

Advocacy: Genetic Alliance, a non-profit group based in Washington, D.C., advocates for patients' rights in genomic health issues and provides information and support. *www.geneticalliance.org*

The Genetics and Public Policy Center, based at Johns Hopkins University in Maryland, works to help policy makers and the public better understand the working and effects of genomic science. Leaders at the center also help promote fair, ethical genomic practices and laws. *www.dnapolicy.org*

Allergy: The American Academy of Allergy, Asthma, and Immunology offers a wide variety of health information, including the genomic aspects of allergic conditions. *www.aaaai.org*

Alzheimer's disease: The Alzheimer's Association provides information on all aspects of this condition, including genetic testing and ongoing gene research. *www.alz.org*

American College of Medical Genetics: This group mostly represents doctors who specialize in gene-related care, but also offers information on current medical policies in the genomic world. *www.acmg.net*

APOE alleles and testing: Lab Tests Online, a non-commercial Web site sponsored by a variety of medical testing companies, offers a thorough overview of possible uses and limits of APOE testing. *www.labtestsonline.org/understanding/analytes/apoe/glance.html*

Asthma: The American Academy of Allergy, Asthma, and Immunology offers a wide variety of health information, including the genomic aspects of asthma. *www.aaaai.org*

Autism: The Autism Society of America provides a wide variety of information and offers family and patient support. *www.autism-society.org*

The Autism Genome Project releases news of its findings to the public through Autism Speaks, a non-profit group that supports autism research. *www.autismspeaks.org*

Behavioral genetics: The official Web site for the Human Genome Project features a good introduction to the study of genes, the brain, behavior, and personality. *www.ornl.gov/sci/techresources/Human_Genome/elsi/behavior.shtml*

Birth defects: The March of Dimes, a leading advocate in this aspect of health care, regularly offers updates on gene research and emerging treatments for infants with genetic ailments. *www.marchofdimes.org*

Blood clots: Through its online health encyclopedia Medline, the National Institutes of Health offers information on a variety of different types of clots, including those with genetic links. *www.nlm.nih.gov/medlineplus/ency/article/001124.htm*

BRCA testing: The National Cancer Institute provides an overview of testing for both *BRCA1* and *BRCA2* mutations. *http://www.cancer.gov/cancertopics/factsheet/Risk/BRCA*

Facing Our Risk of Cancer Empowered, a non-profit advocacy group, focuses on women whose genes give them a greater risk of breast or ovarian cancer. *www.facingourrisk.org*

Breast cancer: Breastcancer.org provides medically reviewed information on all aspects of breast cancer. *www.breastcancer.org*

Susan G. Komen for the Cure, a nationwide nonprofit, provides information, advocacy, and patient support. *cms.komen.org/komen/AboutUs/index.htm*

Cancer: The largest nonprofit related to this condition, the American Cancer Society offers general information, updates on gene research, and patient support. *www.cancer.org*

The National Cancer Institute provides information for both the public and medical professionals, including updates on genetic testing, genomic research, and gene-centered treatments. *www.cancer.gov*

The National Cancer Institute also lets you track the latest work of the Cancer Genome Atlas. *http://cancergenome.nih.gov/index.asp*

Celiac disease: The Celiac Disease Foundation provides a wide range of patient information and support, including dietary guidelines and tips. *www.celiac.org*

Cervical cancer: The National Cancer Institute offers a thorough overview of this condition, including updates on HPV gene tests and vaccines. *http://www.cancer.gov/cancertopics/types/cervical*

Clinical trials: Developed by the National Institutes of Health, this site offers both an overview of how trials work and a database where you can find trials by topic and/or location. *www.clinicaltrials.gov*

Cloning: The official site for the Human Genome Project includes an overview of different types of cloning, practical limitations, and ethical concerns. *www.ornl.gov/sci/techresources/Human_Genome/elsi/cloning.shtml*

Colorectal cancer: The National Cancer Institute offers a thorough overview of this condition, including updates on genetic testing and emerging targeted therapies. *www.cancer.gov/cancertopics/types/colon-and-rectal*

Founded by colon cancer patients, the Colon Cancer Alliance provides a wide range of patient support, as well as information on cancer screening and genetic testing. *www.ccalliance.org*

Cystic fibrosis: The Cystic Fibrosis Foundation offers health information and patient support. *www.cff.org*

The American College of Obstetricians and Gynecologists offers a patient-centered booklet to help people make a decision about cystic fibrosis carrier testing. *www.acog.org/from_home/wellness/cf001.htm*

Depression: The National Institute of Mental Health offers an overview of symptoms, suggestions on treatment and finding help, and updates on research news. *www.nimh.nih.gov/healthinformation/depressionmenu.cfm*

Diabetes: The American Diabetes Association offers a wide range of information and support, including updates on gene research and dietary suggestions. *www.diabetes.org/home.jsp*

Down syndrome: The National Down Syndrome Society website presents information about innovative education, research, and advocacy programs to ensure that people with Down syndrome realize their hopes and dreams. *www.ndss.org*

Keep up with the latest medical recommendations for Down syndrome screening during pregnancy at the Web site for the American College of Obstetricians and Gynecologists. *www.acog.org*

Ethical issues in genomic medicine: The National Human Genome Research Institute presents an overview of ethical issues in genomic care and the way those concerns shape public policy. *www.genome.gov/PolicyEthics*

The official site for the Human Genome Project includes an overview of ethical issues in all aspects of gene science, including genomic medicine. *www.ornl.gov/elsi/elsi.html*

Family medical history: The National Society of Genetic Counselors offers a guide to creating your own family medical history, either with a computer or using pen and paper. *www.nsgc.org*

The U.S. Surgeon General's office offers computerized tools for creating a family medical history either online or through software downloaded to your own computer. *www.hhs.gov/familyhistory*

Here you will find one of many informative family history reviews developed by the respected Mayo Clinic. *http://www.mayoclinic.com/health/medical-history/HQ01707*

Genetic Alliance also offers family history tools, and is developing versions specific to certain ethnic groups. *www.geneticalliance.org*

Federal rules governing genomic medicine: For complex legal reasons, the federal Food and Drug Administration doesn't regulate most genetic tests now in use. But the agency does approve new genomic treatments, and also lets patients file complaints about drugs and medical devices. *www.fda.gov*

Fragile X syndrome: The National Fragile X Foundation offers general information and support for patients and families. *www.fragilex.org*

Gene overviews: Genetics Home Reference, published by the National Library of Medicine, offers a thorough overview of genes and human DNA, along with in-depth looks at how specific genes affect health. *ghr.nlm.nih.gov*

The National Human Genome Research Institute provides a detailed explanation of genes, as well as updates on new genomic research. *www.genome.gov*

From England, the nonprofit Wellcome Trust provides thorough background on human genes and frequent updates on gene treatments and research. *www.genome.wellcome.ac.uk*

The University of Utah operates this fun and informative site that not only explains genes but shows how they work in various aspects of medicine. *http://learn.genetics.utah.edu*

Gene maps: At the official site for the Human Genome Project, you'll find detailed maps of each human chromosome, explaining the location of particular mutations and their health effects. *www.ornl.gov/sci/techresources/Human_Genome/posters/chromosome/hbb.shtml*

Gene therapy: The official site for the Human Genome Project includes an overview of different types of gene therapy.
www.ornl.gov/sci/techresources/Human_Genome/medicine/genetherapy.shtml

Gene vocabulary: To learn the meaning of a gene-related term, visit the glossary operated by the National Human Genome Research Institute. *www.genome.gov/10002096*

Genetic counseling: The National Society of Genetic Counselors not only represents this group of professionals, but offers a wide variety of public information on working with and finding a genetic counselor. *www.nsgc.org*

Genetic discrimination: The National Human Genome Research Institute provides an overview of discrimination issues and tracks some of the legal reforms aimed at preventing discrimination. *www.genome.gov/10002077*

The nonprofit Council for Responsible Genetics actively promotes genetic fairness and promotes public discussion of privacy and discrimination concerns. *www.gene-watch.org*

Genetic Alliance leads lobbying efforts in Washington, D.C., for stronger laws against genetic discrimination. *www.geneticalliance.org*

Genetic illness: Genetics Home Reference, published by the National Library of Medicine, offers in-depth looks at specific gene-related conditions. *ghr.nlm.nih.gov*

Genetic inheritance: A massive library linking specific genes and their variations to behavioral and health issues, the searchable site Online Mendelian Inheritance in Man offers detailed histories and descriptions of gene discoveries. The information on this site is often technical and science-heavy, but if you want the full scientific story on an inherited health issue, OMIM is the place to go. *www.ncbi.nlm.nih.gov/entrez/query.fcgi?db=OMIM*

Genetic privacy: The official site for the Human Genome Project provides a chronological overview of privacy laws and ongoing efforts to change them. *www.ornl.gov/sci/techresources/Human_Genome/elsi/legislat.shtml*

Genetic Alliance leads lobbying efforts in Washington, D.C., for stronger laws to protect genetic privacy. *www.geneticalliance.org*

Genetic testing: GeneTests, a nonprofit information service, provides background on hundreds of genetic tests and updates on tests in development. *www.genetests.org*

This non-commercial information service explains how a wide variety of medical tests work, including genetic tests. *www.labtestsonline.org*

The official site for the Human Genome Project includes an overview of pros and cons of testing. *www.ornl.gov/sci/techresources/Human_Genome/medicine/genetest.shtml*

Heart health: In addition to general background information and prevention and treatment ideas, the American Heart Association also offers information on genes related to cardiac care. *www.americanheart.org*

Get updates on healthy cholesterol levels, testing, and treatment options at this site operated by the National Cholesterol Education Program. *www.nhlbi.nih.gov/chd*

Health professional education: The National Coalition for Health Professional Education in Genetics develops and offers education and training in all aspects of genomics for a wide variety of health professionals working in primary care. *www.nchpeg.org*

Hemochromatosis (Iron Overload): Started by a woman with a family history of this disease, the American Hemochromatosis Society offers information, advice, and patient support. *www.americanhs.org*

Hemophilia: The National Hemophilia Foundation focuses on helping to find treatments and cures for blood clotting disorders. *www.hemophilia.org*

Human Genome Project: The official site for the federally funded Human Genome Project offers information on genes, the science behind the decoding of the human genome, and how our genome's mapping is shaping health and society. *www.ornl.gov/sci/techresources/Human_Genome/home.shtml*

Long QT syndrome: For people interested in learning more about long QT, this site offers a helpful blend of scientific background and real-life experience. Although the site is based in Switzerland, it's primary language is English. *www.qtsyndrome.ch/about.html*

The Mayo Clinic provides thorough medical background information on long QT syndrome. *www.mayoclinic.com/health/long-qt-syndrome/DS00434*

Lung cancer: The American Lung Association includes information on lung cancer among its library of respiratory health information, and also features phone numbers and email addresses where you can ask questions of a health care professional. *www.lungusa.org*

Leukemia and lymphoma: The Leukemia and Lymphoma Society includes frequent news on genomic care among its background information, treatment updates, and patient support. *www.leukemia.org*

Newborn screening: In its work against birth defects, the March of Dimes advocates for more comprehensive newborn screening and helps expectant parents choose the most thorough testing program possible. *www.marchofdimes.org*

Nutrigenomics: As part of its scientific work with genes and diet research into The Center for Excellence in Nutritional Genomics at the University of California at Davis offers a wide range of public information on specific conditions and ongoing research. *nutrigenomics.ucdavis.edu*

Ovarian cancer: The National Cancer Institute presents a thorough overview, including statistics, treatment news, and information on finding clinical trials. *www.cancer.gov/cancertopics/types/ovarian*

Pancreatic cancer: The Pancreatic Cancer Action Network (PanCAN) provides information for patients and health care professionals and is working to support research efforts. *http://www.pancan.org/index.html*

Personal genome sequencing: Based at Harvard, genomic expert George Church is leading the science and effects of personal genomes and makes all its findings public. *arep.med.harvard.edu/PGP*

This personal blog, created by a genetic testing professional, tracks news in all aspects of personal gene sequencing. *www.thepersonalgenome.com*

Personalized medicine: The National Institutes of Health offers an online booklet detailing ongoing work to match medicines to your genes. *publications.nigms.nih.gov/medbydesign*

Pervasive development disorders: Going beyond autism, the National Institute of Mental Health offers information on the full range of autism-related conditions. *www.nimh.nih.gov/publicat/autism.cfm*

Preimplantation genetic diagnosis (PGD): The nonprofit Center for Genetics and Society offers information on the science and ethical debates surrounding PGD. *www.genetics-and-society.org/technologies/other/pgd.html*

Prenatal testing: Lab Tests Online, a non-commercial Web site sponsored by a variety of medical testing companies, offers a thorough overview of all prenatal testing, including predictive and diagnostic screening. *www.labtestsonline.org/understanding/conditions/pregnancy-12.html*

Prostate cancer: Visit this National Cancer Institute page for medical background, treatment news, and the latest on clinical trials. *www.cancer.gov/cancertopics/types/prostate*

This nonprofit provides both patient support and funding for prostate cancer research. *www.prostatecancerfoundation.org*

RNA interference (RNAi): NOVA, a leading public television science program, offers both an explanation of how RNAi works and outlines a few of its possible medical uses. *www.pbs.org/wgbh/nova/sciencenow/3210/02.html*

Sickle cell anemia: Genetics Home Reference offers an easy-to-understand explanation of how a gene mutation drives sickle cell disease, along with links to health and treatment information. *ghr.nlm.nih.gov/condition=sicklecelldisease*

Single nucleotide polymorphisms (SNPs): The National Center for Biotechnology Information offers an easy-to-understand look at SNPs and the roles they play in our health. *www.ornl.gov/sci/techresources/Human_Genome/faq/snps.shtml*

Stem cell overview: The National Institutes of Health provides an overview that blends scientific background with the last national policies on stem cells and background on ethical concerns. *stemcells.nih.gov*

Stem cell advocacy: Pushing for more federal support for human embryonic stem cell research, the Coalition for the Advancement of Medical Research represents people with a range of health issues that might be improved by stem cell therapies. *www.camradvocacy.org*

Many conservative religious groups oppose embryonic stem cell research and lobby against it, including the Catholic Church, whose explanation of opposition efforts reflects the views of many stem cell research opponents. *www.americancatholic.org/News/StemCell*

Telomeres: The Genetic Science Learning Center at the University of Utah offers a detailed explanation of how telomeres protect your DNA, as well as how any damage to them might affect health and aging. *learn.genetics.utah.edu/features/telomeres*

INDEX